T0162267

T'AI CHI

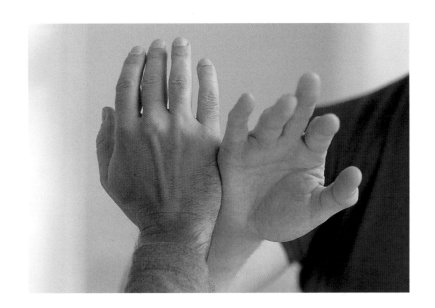

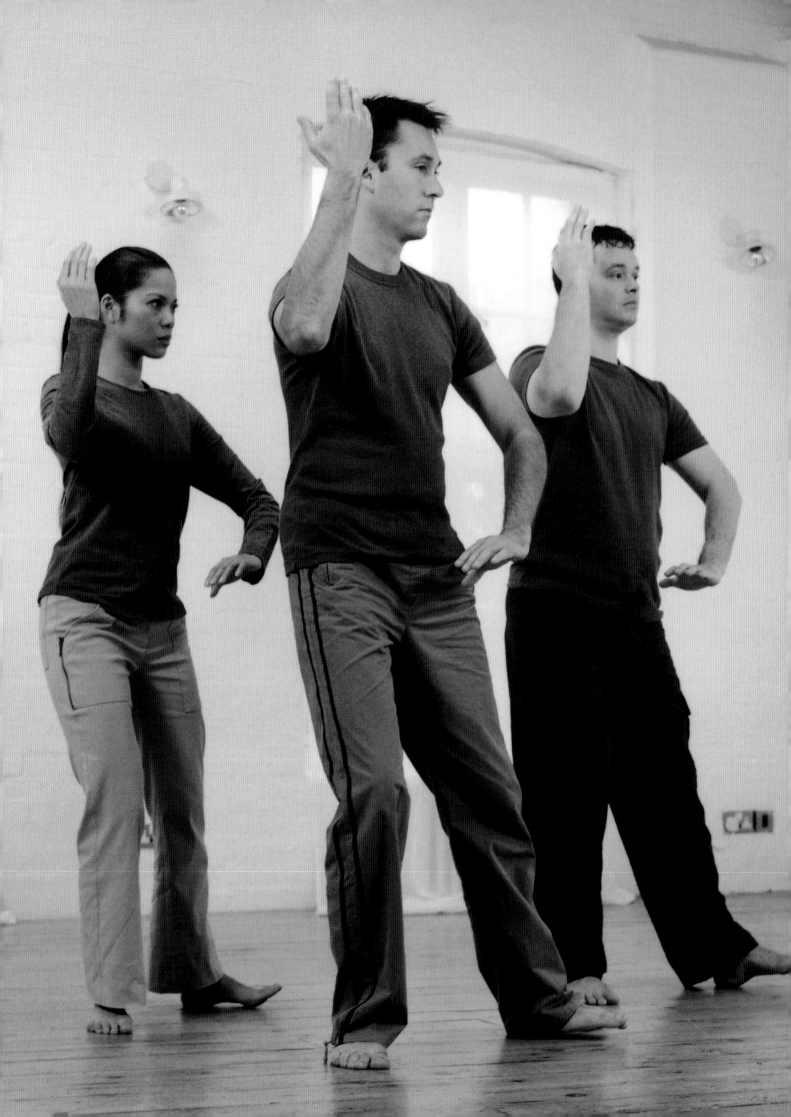

T'AI CHI

ANCIENT PHYSICAL SYSTEMS FOR CREATING INNER
HARMONY AND EQUILIBRIUM

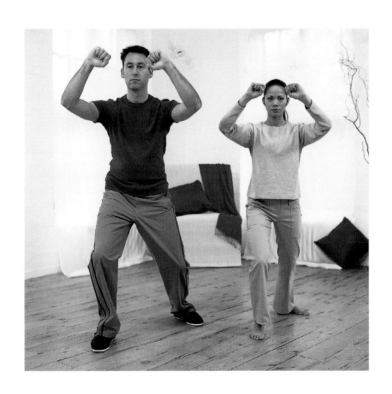

Andrew Popovic

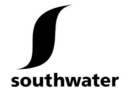

southwater

TThis edition is published by Southwater,
an imprint of Anness Publishing Ltd
Hermes House, 88-89 Blackfriars Road, London SE1 8HA
tel. 020 7401 2077; fax 020 7633 9499
www.southwaterbooks.com; www.annesspublishing.com

© Anness Publishing Ltd 2004, 2010

UK agent: The Manning Partnership Ltd, 6 The Old Dairy, Melcombe Road,
Bath BA2 3LR; tel. 01225 478444; fax 01225 478440;
sales@manning-partnership.co.uk
UK distributor: Book Trade Services; tel. 0116 2759086; fax 0116 2759090;
uksales@booktradeservices.com; exportsales@booktradeservices.com
North American agent/distributor: National Book Network,
4501 Forbes Boulevard, Suite 200, Lanham, MD 20706; tel. 301 459 3366;
fax 301 429 5746; www.nbnbooks.com
Australian agent/distributor: Pan Macmillan Australia, Level 18,
St Martins Tower, 31 Market St, Sydney, NSW 2000;
tel. 1300 135 113; fax 1300 135 103; customer.service@macmillan.com.au
New Zealand agent/distributor: David Bateman Ltd, 30 Tarndale Grove,
Off Bush Road, Albany, Auckland; tel. (09) 415 7664; fax (09) 415 8892

All rights reserved. No part of this publication may be reproduced, stored in
a retrieval system, or transmitted in any way or by any means, electronic,
mechanical, photocopying, recording or otherwise, without the prior written
permission of the copyright holder.

Publisher Joanna Lorenz
Editorial Director Helen Sudell
Executive Editor Joanne Rippin
Copy Editor Beverley Jollands
Designer Nigel Partridge
Photography Clare Park
Production Manager Darren Price
Editorial Reader Penelope Goodare

ETHICAL TRADING POLICY
Because of our ongoing ecological investment programme, you,
as our customer, can have the pleasure and reassurance of
knowing that a tree is being cultivated on your behalf to
naturally replace the materials used to make the book you are
holding. For further information about this scheme, go to
www.annesspublishing.com/trees

The author and publishers have made every effort to ensure that all
instructions contained within this book are accurate and safe, and cannot
accept liability for any resulting injury, damage or loss to persons or
property, however it may arise. If you do have any special needs or
problems, consult your doctor or another health professional. This book
cannot replace medical consultation and should be used in conjunction
with professional advice. You should not attempt t'ai chi without training
from a properly qualified practitioner.

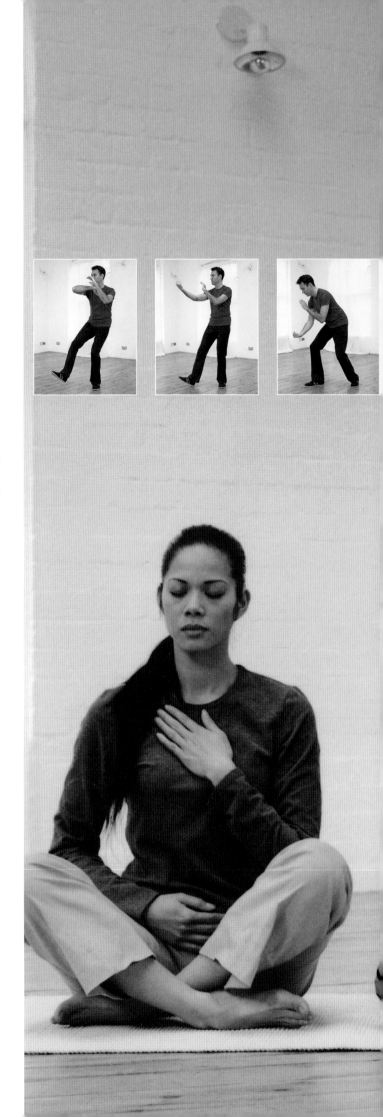

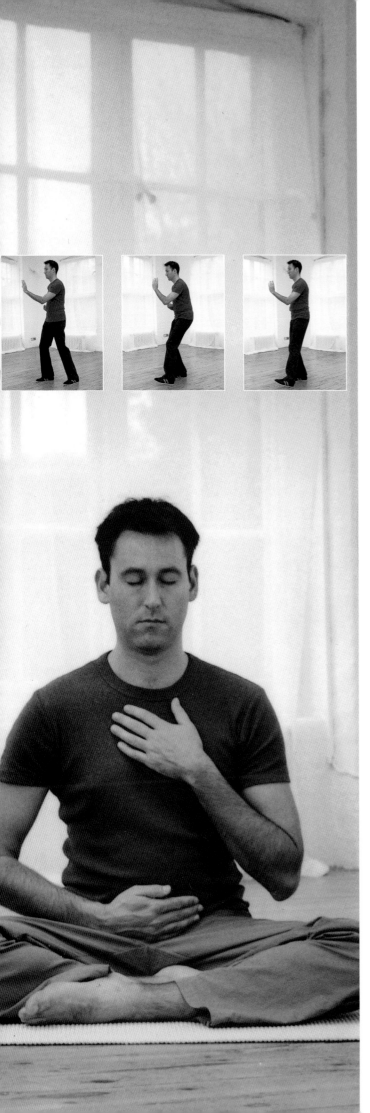

Contents

Introduction

T'ai chi is an art of balance: physical, energetic, mental and emotional balance. T'ai chi began in ancient China, and is known as an internal art – meaning an art of self-development. From a t'ai chi perspective, self-development means gaining robust health, a balanced emotional life and clarity of mind, and evolving spiritually. The practice of t'ai chi consists of a set of smoothly flowing movements called the "form". The form is normally performed at a relatively slow pace, allowing for the gradual release of tension in your body and mind; the healing of physical injuries and imbalances; and the opening and energizing of the energetic channels and centres of the body. The structure of the movements of the t'ai chi form are designed to enhance the energetic flows within your body – and they also happen to be very beautiful and graceful. Although as a beginning t'ai chi student one's main focus is on learning the external movements, or "form", as one progresses it is possible to focus more on the internal aspects of t'ai chi, including the use of one's mind to move and transform one's chi energy. This is where

Below The practise of t'ai chi simultaneously balances the physical, energetic, mental and emotional aspects of your being

many of the deeper benefits of t'ai chi are to be found. In fact, t'ai chi can become a very powerful form of moving meditation, as well as an ideal health practice.

T'ai chi has its roots in the Taoist tradition, whose origins date back 5,000 years. Later in the book we will look more fully at the origins and theories that underlie t'ai chi. Fundamentally, t'ai chi is concerned with the principle of balancing yin and yang – the mutually complementary aspects of existence that can be applied to all concepts, such as night and day, female and male, etc. The diagram Taoists use to illustrate this theory is known as the t'ai chi symbol. It shows yin changing into yang, and vice versa, in a never-ending cycle, and the totality of the two, and therefore the totality of existence, is represented by the entire symbol – hence t'ai chi or "Great Ultimate". The full name of this art is in fact t'ai chi chuan. The word chuan means "fist" – and this hints at its martial origins.

T'ai chi is most commonly practised purely for its health and self-development benefits, but it is also a martial art, and a highly effective one. Ancient China was a dangerous place, and self-defence was an essential skill, not a sport or pastime. Inseparable from the martial nature of t'ai chi are

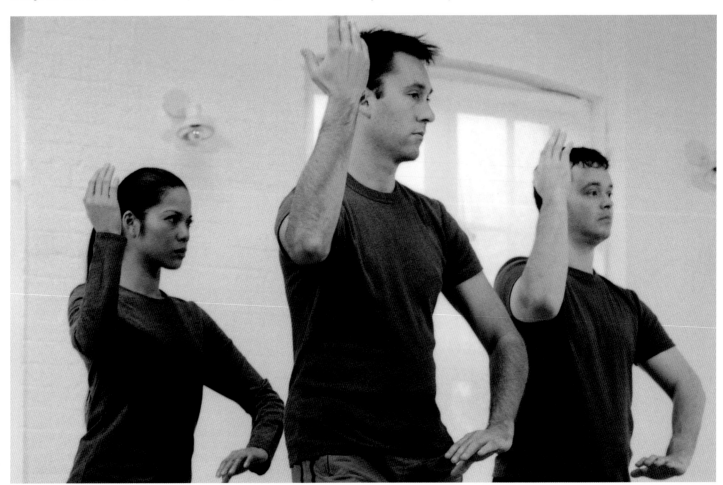

its self-development aspects. In fact, t'ai chi simply does not work as a high-level martial art without at least some of the self-development aspects being accomplished. However, you can use t'ai chi effectively as a self-development tool without ever engaging in martial practice. For the vast majority of people who practise t'ai chi today, this is the case. Becoming relaxed, healthy and balanced is a more important survival skill for most people in the modern world than becoming a proficient fighter. You are much more likely to die from a stress-related disease than be killed by a criminal. In this sense t'ai chi is a truly modern self-defence art – defence against the very real enemy of stress-related illness.

WHY LEARN T'AI CHI?

T'ai chi operates on several levels simultaneously: the physical, the energetic and the mental/emotional. Most people in the modern world (and probably in any culture) suffer from some form of physical imbalance or injury – for instance, back and neck pain, which is almost epidemic in developed societies, where many people lead sedentary, desk-bound lives. T'ai chi allows for the release and healing of physical tensions and injuries – over time it has the

potential to completely eliminate back, neck and joint problems. This in itself is a compelling reason to learn the art of t'ai chi, but another, perhaps even more compelling, reason to practise t'ai chi is stress. Levels of stress have become almost intolerable for many people around the world. The only effective antidote to stress is to learn to relax, but this is often easier said than done. T'ai chi offers an enjoyable and engaging way to relax both your body and your mind – without giving up your existing life. With some initial effort to learn t'ai chi, and as little as 15 minutes' practice a day, you can greatly reduce the levels of stress you experience. More practice brings even greater calmness and balance in the midst of an often chaotic world. With no special equipment or space needed, most people could easily perform a t'ai chi form in their living room, making it ideal for city-dwellers.

For those who have a deeper interest in meditation and spiritual practice, t'ai chi offers a solid foundation for these practices, as it allows for the release of emotional tensions,

Below T'ai chi originated in ancient China and has since spread throughout the world due to its ability to benefit all types of people.

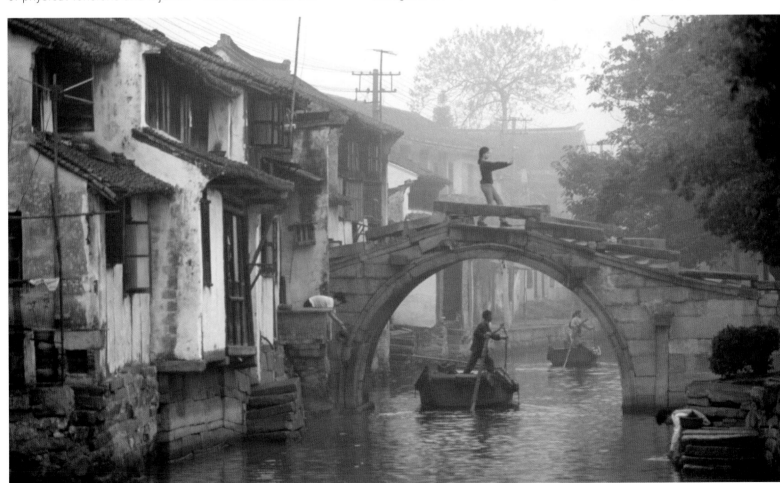

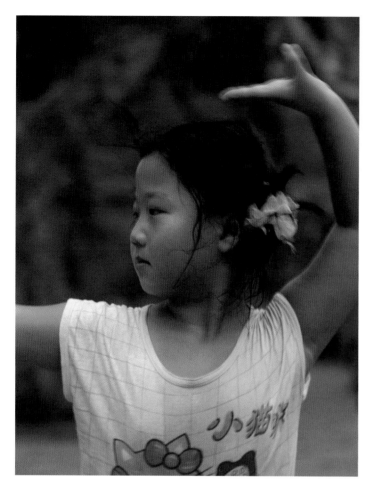

Left T'ai chi appeals to all ages, from 7 to 70, and beyond. It is one of the most powerful longevity practices in existence.

Right T'ai chi is enjoyed equally by men and women. It does not rely on strength or aggression, but instead cultivates relaxation.

and develops stillness of mind within the practitioner – essential prerequisites for deeper meditation practices. Above all, t'ai chi works at the level of your energy – what the Chinese call "chi". Chi is the living energy that circulates through your body, and it is what makes you alive – a dead body has no chi circulating through it. The Chinese medical art of acupuncture works directly with your chi to release blockage and balance the flow of this energy through specific pathways in the body in order to cure the imbalances that lead to illness. By a combination of specific movements and mental intention in t'ai chi, you can move chi around your own body, in the process clearing blockages in, and balancing, your energy, as well as increasing your energetic reserves (relating to your energetic centre known as the lower tantien). This will in turn affect your physical body, allowing it to relax and heal itself – and it will affect your mind, because when your energy is balanced and relaxed, so is your mind.

Sometimes t'ai chi is referred to as a mind–body art, and this is a very appropriate term, because ideally there is no separation between the two when practising (in fact, the term could be mind–energy–body, as t'ai chi works on all these levels at the same time). With its emphasis on finding stillness in the midst of movement – both your own movement and that of the world around you – t'ai chi offers a practical way to greatly enhance your day-to-day experience of living in this often turbulent world, while also helping you evolve as a person and find greater happiness and peace within yourself.

HOW TO GET THE MOST FROM THIS BOOK

Learning t'ai chi can be both simple and complex. The essence of t'ai chi is simple; the methods used to get to an understanding of that essence can seem complex. T'ai chi is about feeling rather than thinking. It is possible to collect a lot of intellectual knowledge about t'ai chi, without really penetrating the essence of what it is to do t'ai chi. The real benefits of t'ai chi come from integrating its core principles within your being. In this sense, simplicity is best. This book contains fundamental information, t'ai chi principles, and exercises that, if applied, can give you a taste of this extraordinary art, and help you gain some genuine understanding and experience of t'ai chi.

In one sense this book is linear – you can start at the beginning, passing through an overview of t'ai chi and the Taoist tradition it stems from, then read the in-depth chapters on the different aspects of t'ai chi. After that, there is a practical section giving you exercises to prepare you for learning the t'ai chi form itself, and to help you relax and release tension in your body. Then there is a complete t'ai chi short form to learn, followed by discussion on some of the deeper aspects of t'ai chi practice, including the martial aspects of t'ai chi.

However, learning t'ai chi and developing your practice is not really a linear process. As you progress, you will return to information and exercises that you passed through previously, relearning and reinterpreting them many times in the light of your developing understanding and ability. This is one of the reasons why t'ai chi is truly a life-long journey – if you persevere and practise, you will never find it becomes boring or limited. Instead it becomes deeper and more mysterious – taking you on a fascinating and rewarding journey into your own nature. The Taoists say that you have to learn something three times before you truly start to understand it. Try reading this book three times over, before starting to practise. Absorb the information in this book first, and you will progress faster. Once on your way, you will find it useful to revisit parts of the book, understanding previously read material in a new light.

We need to be patient with ourselves when learning t'ai chi, and realistic about the speed at which we can naturally develop. If we do this, we will progress much faster than if we place unreasonable demands and expectations on ourselves. This is for one simple reason – we will be more relaxed. T'ai chi is all about deep relaxation – this is where the real skill lies. A key phrase traditionally used in learning the Taoist internal arts translates as "more or less". One more or less learns something and more or less does it correctly. With time and practice, and with a relaxed attitude

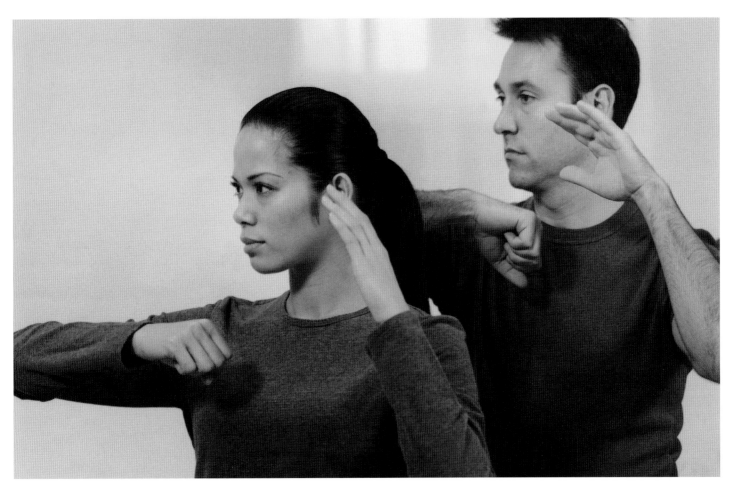

to one's progress, it becomes more rather than less. But "more or less" implies something very important: you will never do t'ai chi perfectly, just "more" rather than "less". Trying to be perfect is an automatic recipe for failure, so instead, try to relax and enjoy what you can do in the present time.

CHINESE TERMS

The Chinese language does not easily translate into Western languages: it is highly metaphorical and is based on ideograms (pictorial representations of words or concepts) rather than phonetic symbols. Multiple transliterations exist of almost all Chinese terms (there are three separate systems of transliteration in general use). This book uses the transliterations that are either the easiest to pronounce, and closest (in English) to the Chinese pronunciation, or the most widely established transliterations of a particular term. For instance, t'ai chi would be more accurately transliterated as "t'ai jee" – the chi/"jee" in t'ai chi is not the same word as the chi (pronounced "chee") in chi gung. However, the transliteration "t'ai chi" is so universal that is has been retained. Tantien is pronounced "dandien", but again, tantien is used almost universally. Chi gung can be transliterated as "chi kung" or "qi gong", but neither of these is close to the correct pronunciation, and since there is no universally used transliteration, in this case "chi gung" has been used as it is closest to the correct pronunciation. This approach is designed to minimize confusion for the reader.

HOW TO BEGIN

The first two chapters of the book, although not practical sections, do contain important concepts that relate directly to your t'ai chi practice, and you will find these essential to your deeper understanding of t'ai chi. As you progress, you may find it useful to re-read those chapters, and incorporate those concepts into your practice.

To start learning t'ai chi itself, spend as much time as possible running through the exercises set out in the "Preparation" chapter. The sections titled "T'ai Chi Principles" and "Relaxing and Releasing" contain the essential information you will need to start moving in a "t'ai chi" manner. The section on "Taoist Breathing" contains exercises to help still your mind and relax your entire body – an essential t'ai chi skill. The section on "Cloud Hands" contains a complete chi gung exercise that embodies the essence of t'ai chi. This will help you develop your t'ai chi skills before, during and after learning the form.

In "The Wu Style Short Form" a complete t'ai chi short form is set out, clearly illustrated and described in order to guide you through the sequence of postures. These movements use principles that you will have already learned from the previous chapter. In keeping with the circular nature of this learning process, you will find it useful to refer back to "Preparation" as you progress through learning the form. "Taking it Further" contains more advanced information, including push hands techniques, pulsing joints, and exercises for meditation to help you to develop your practice and integrate it into your entire lifestyle.

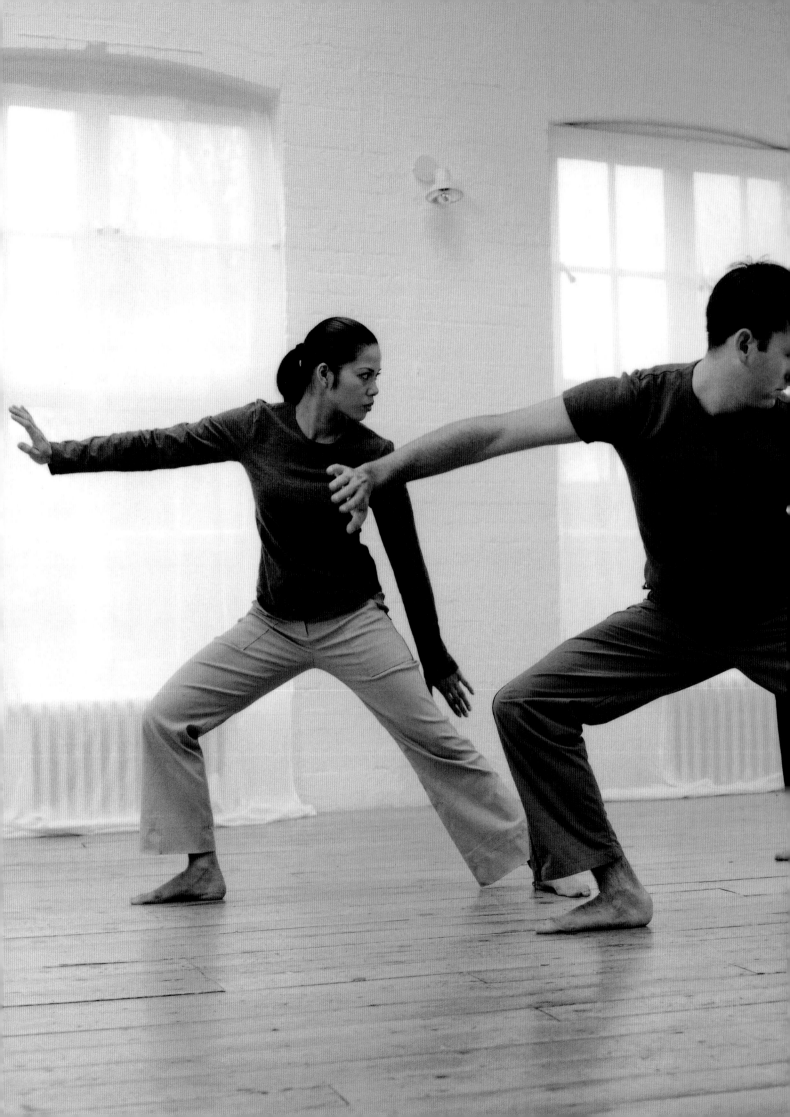

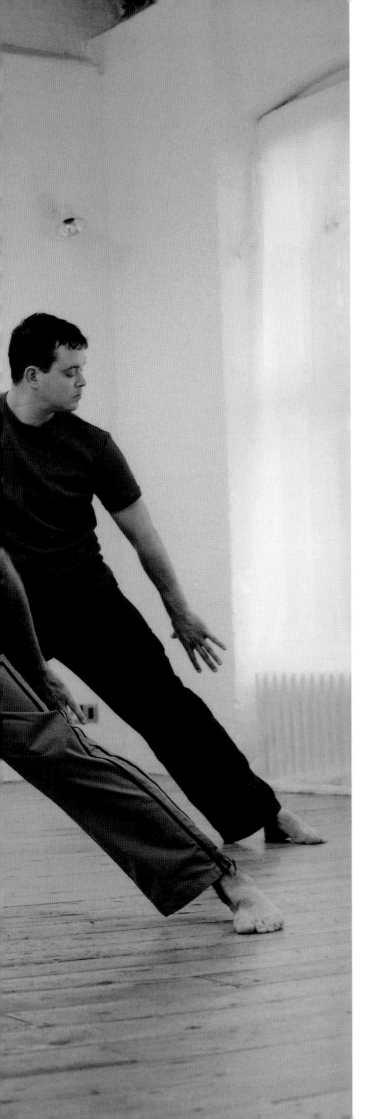

T'ai Chi in Context

This chapter looks at the origins and place of t'ai chi in relation to the other Taoist arts of China. Understanding how t'ai chi developed and evolved and how it relates to the other Taoist arts can lead to a much deeper understanding of what it is you are seeking to learn and practise. T'ai chi does not stand alone; it embodies aspects of, and is intrinsically linked to, all the Taoist arts and sciences, such as other Taoist internal martial arts, chi gung (energy work), meditation, feng shui (geomancy), Chinese astrology and Chinese medicine. The common thread running through all these arts is an understanding of energy, called chi. This energy underlies all manifestation in the universe – solid matter merely being a very condensed form of chi energy. By understanding chi we can begin fully to understand ourselves.

The Taoist Tradition

A Taoist (pronounced "Daoist") is a person who "follows the Tao". Tao means "way" or "path" in Chinese, and in this context it means the way of the universe and all existence. Following the Tao means living in total harmony with the universe and understanding the nature of reality. True Taoism is a spiritual tradition, the origins of which date back at least 5,000 years in China. Never an organized religion, it is rather a personal spiritual path.

The Taoists were never great in number, yet they had an enormous influence on Chinese thought, art and science: much of the cultural heritage that we would identify as being characteristically Chinese is of Taoist origin. They were the originators of Chinese medicine, calligraphy and art, feng shui, chi gung and the internal arts, astrology and cosmology, and traditional music and theatre. Taoist sages usually avoided entanglement in politics and government, but they were often the guiding light behind the wiser Chinese rulers. The most prosperous and peaceful periods of Chinese history have usually coincided with a strong Taoist influence.

Although Taoism had existed in some form for several thousand years before his birth, the concept is commonly attributed to the sage Lao-tzu (570–490 BC). He held the very important post of Imperial Librarian and was known during his lifetime as a great Taoist master. As an old man, he withdrew from worldly affairs, renounced his position and

Below Lao-tzu, the founder of Taoism, seen here seated on his buffalo, and followed by a disciple.

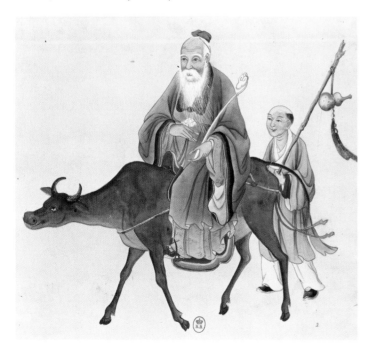

set off for Tibet riding a water buffalo. A border guard, himself a Taoist, insisted that Lao-tzu leave behind a manuscript of the most essential Taoist teachings before he disappeared from the world. Lao-tzu agreed to this and wrote what is known as the Tao Te Ching or the "Book of the Way and its Virtue".

The Tao Te Ching was the first book to be written on Taoism, which until then had been a purely oral tradition, hence Lao-tzu's reputation as its "originator". This short book, consisting of 81 verses, contains the essence of the ancient Taoist "water method" tradition (the metaphor of water is repeatedly used in the text). This emphasizes the dissolving of all tension in one's being, in contrast to the "fire method", which advocates making things happen.

TAOIST BELIEFS

Taoists hold that the source of all existence is emptiness. From this, two opposite and complementary aspects of energy arise: yin and yang. These two principles cannot exist independently of one another, just as you cannot define darkness (yin) without the concept of light (yang), or female (yin) without male (yang). Just as they are mutually dependent, yin and yang contain the essence of one another within themselves, shown in the t'ai chi symbol by the small dot of the opposite colour within each half. They constantly change into one another, as night changes into day and back again in an endless cycle, and this is also shown in the symbol: as one decreases the other increases, and as each reaches its maximum it starts to change into its opposite. For example, after midday, which is considered fully yang, there is a change to yin as the sun starts to descend. Midnight is fully yin: after that point yang energy increases.

The t'ai chi symbol (shown right) is perhaps the most famous symbol in the world and is an elegant way of describing the nature of the universe. "T'ai chi" is really another way of saying "Tao" – the totality of existence.

Right An elderly t'ai chi practitioner cultivating "stillness within movement, and movement within stillness". The deeper aspects of t'ai chi embody the principles of Taoist spiritual practice.

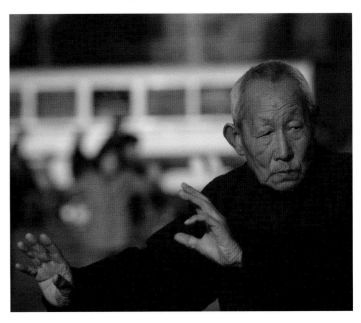

> Mysteriously formed,
> Born before heaven and earth.
> In the silence and the void,
> Standing alone and unchanging,
> Ever present and in motion;
> It is the mother of the ten thousand things.
> It has no name. Call it the Way [Tao].
> Lao-tzu, Tao Te Ching

THE FIVE ELEMENTS

Following the division of yin and yang energy out of emptiness, five distinct phases of energy – known as the Five Elements – are formed. These are Metal, Water, Wood, Fire and Earth. Just as everything can be described in terms of yin and yang, it can also be described in terms of the Five Elements. In the cycle of the seasons, for instance, midsummer has the quality of Fire, late summer of Earth, autumn of Metal, winter of Water and spring of Wood. Each element (and each season in this case) generates the next, in what is known as the Generation Cycle. The names of the elements are essentially ways of describing a particular type of energy: Wood, for example, has the quality of expanding energy, or growth. Five Element theory is fundamental to Chinese medicine. Each of the body's organs embodies a characteristic element – for instance, the heart is Fire, and the kidneys are Water – and people exhibit more or less of each element in their behaviour and physical make-up.

From the Five Elements are formed the Ten Thousand Things (symbolizing the multitude of objects found in the universe). This concept forms a complete description of how the universe unfolds out of nothingness – a description that has been supported in modern times by quantum physics.

THE I CHING

Another very famous Taoist book, the I Ching or "Book of Changes", further describes the universe in terms of patterns of yin and yang, represented by solid or broken lines. These are put together in groups of three to make eight symbols called trigrams. Together these are known as the ba gua, and they are often shown grouped around a t'ai chi symbol, further describing the process of change from yin to yang and back again. The eight trigrams are then combined in pairs to make 64 hexagrams, which represent all possible changes of energy in the universe.

Taoists say that if one understands the I Ching, then one truly understands the nature of existence. It can be used on many levels: for help in forecasting future events, for advice on how to deal with our current situation and as a key to understanding the universe and our place in it.

The essence of Taoism lies in its understanding of the nature of existence or, as Taoists would say, reality. Yin/yang theory, the ba gua, the I Ching and the Five Elements are all ways of describing this reality. Its source is the mysterious, unknowable Tao, the non-dual state of being beyond even the concept of yin and yang. During the Chinese Cultural Revolution in the 1960s, many Taoists went into hiding or were killed. Taoism was one of the "Olds", the traditional Chinese cultural values that Mao Tse-tung wanted to wipe out. Despite this, Taoism survives as a living tradition.

OTHER CHINESE TRADITIONS

There have of course been other spiritual and philosophical traditions in China, most notably Confucianism and Buddhism. Confucianism – named after Confucius, the Latinized name of the scholar Kung Fu-tzu (551–479 BC) – was very concerned with the role of society and man's place in it (women's roles were strictly defined and limited, whereas the Taoists considered women entirely equal to men). Many Taoist sages, including Lao-tzu himself and another famous master, Chuang-tzu, were openly critical of Confucianism. They felt that Confucianism's obsession with the structure and rules of society took humanity further away from a state of natural harmony and simplicity. Nevertheless, Chinese society to this day is largely Confucian in its attitudes; perhaps this is simply a reflection of the overall Chinese character.

Arriving in China from India in 520 AD, Buddhism was so strongly influenced by the non-gradual Taoist approach to enlightenment that it became a distinct form known as Chan Buddhism. This form later reached Japan, where "Chan" was translated as "Zen".

Another tradition worth mentioning is Neo-Taoism, which arose around the 3rd century AD. While its philosophy was similar to ancient Taoism, it was much more concerned with sorcery, ritual and religious structure. The practices of this tradition are generally more of the "Fire" nature than those used by the ancient Taoists in the "Water" tradition.

Taoist Self-development

The Taoist world view, while fascinating as a philosophy, is not simply a body of intellectual knowledge. It provides the basis for a complete system of self-development that has been tried and tested over millennia. Human nature is no different now from the way it was in ancient China. The Taoist system of self-development views all human beings as essentially the same, subject to the same physical and mental constraints.

Becoming free of the constraints that limit human potential is the very essence of Taoist practice. It is not too bold to say that Taoist self-development is about personal evolution. How far you choose to travel along that path is a personal decision: you may be interested in developing balanced and robust health, or wish to become free of disturbing emotions or to move into the realm of spiritual practice. Taoists maintain that these choices are up to the individual and that no other person has a right to impose them – in other words, everyone has the right to determine the course of their own life.

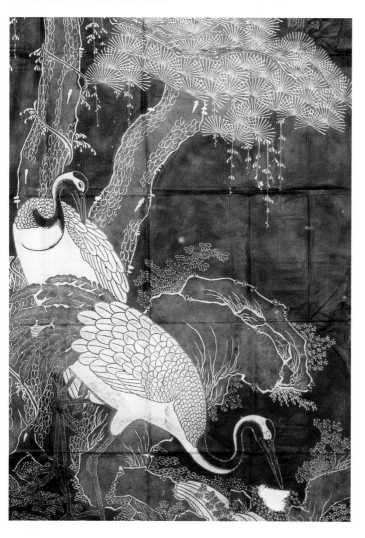

THE MIND OF TAO

Taoism sees humankind as an integral part of the universe, in a harmonious relationship with heaven and earth – yin and yang. Human beings come from the joining of yin and yang. On a physical level we can see this is true: we are the result of the union of male and female potential. However, most human beings rarely experience a state of total integration and harmony. From the earliest times, Taoists sought to transcend the physical, energetic and spiritual separation of human beings from the rest of the universe, and reintegrate with all existence.

Taoism sees the problems we suffer as the result of a loss of this integration. Instead of doing what is natural and appropriate, and therefore beneficial to ourselves, we act in ways that unsettle the body, energy and mind. This causes problems ranging from physical ailments to mental and emotional turmoil, and takes us further away from understanding our true nature and our part in the universe. The Taoists contrast the human mind with the "mind of Tao", which in this context is wisdom, and the human mind represents confusion, or lack of wisdom and clarity. Since everything is Tao, we naturally possess the mind of Tao, but we are preoccupied with the human mind. Taoist practice is about opening ourselves up to, and developing, this potential until we are living with the mind of Tao. This is the state of enlightenment. Along the path to this state, we can learn to live more freely, more healthily, more joyfully.

Ancient Taoist tradition considers that since we are essentially "natural" it is only tensions that stop us enjoying this state. These tensions can exist on many levels, and the tradition talks specifically about eight distinct levels, or "bodies". They range from the physical body through progressively more subtle levels of energy (chi, emotional, mental, psychic, causal, the ego) to the "body of the Tao". These are all aspects of our intrinsic make-up. The tensions that may exist in all these bodies limit our potential and our enjoyment of life. The most obvious example would be a stiff

Left Cranes and pine trees are popular Taoist symbols of the long life and spiritual development they believe is to be gained by sexual and meditative practices, including the practice of t'ai chi.

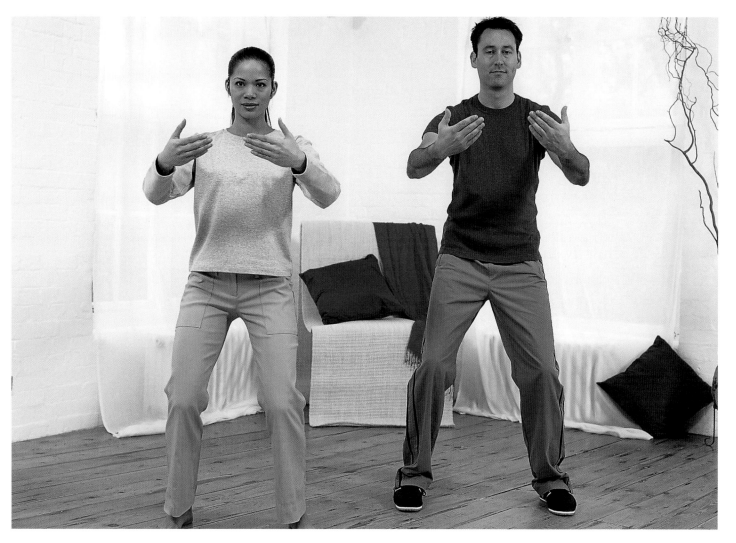

neck or back – tension in the physical body – while we may all experience tension in the emotional body as anger, frustration or depression, or in the mental body as worry.

BECOMING SOONG

In order to overcome such problems we have to release these tensions and become "soong". This Chinese word has no exact translation, but loosely means "unbound". The analogy used is of slitting open a bag of coins and allowing the coins to tumble out freely. It conveys a sense of effortlessly relaxing and letting go. When we do this, our tensions dissolve, and this is what Taoist self-development is about: becoming free of tensions and constraints in the physical body, the mind and emotions. The metaphor of dissolving tension and blockage is at the heart of the water tradition in Taoism.

Since the physical body is the easiest to become aware of and to work with, Taoist self-development practice always starts here. However, the chi body is very closely associated with it. In order to effect change in the physical body, we need to work simultaneously with chi, hence the practices known as chi gung, or "energy work". These release tensions in the physical and chi bodies through physical positions, movements, breathing and mental intent. The benefits are robust health, ample energy and a calm, clear mind. By definition, t'ai chi is a chi gung practice.

Above This chi gung standing practice, known as zhan zhuang, or "standing like a tree", is a powerful method of developing energy.

As your practice develops, you will increasingly access the more subtle levels of your being, such as the emotional and mental bodies, and release tensions at those levels. This feeds back to the chi and physical bodies and you become more relaxed and comfortable. Conversely, mental and emotional tension invariably cause physical tension. You may find it useful to practise meditation, which continues the process of releasing tension, but at the more subtle levels. Its potential benefits are very great, including becoming free of mental and emotional tensions that may have existed for many years.

Taoism has developed many techniques, but all are aimed at achieving this natural state of being soong. The Taoists often refer to babies and very small children as a perfect example of this state: their bodies are relaxed and full of energy, their minds are clear and unconditioned, their emotions relate only to present events, not to past issues or future worries. Regaining the naturalness of a baby while retaining the developed mind of an adult is seen as the ideal. It is the mental and emotional conditioning and physical tension accumulated from early childhood that Taoists seek to become free of, allowing their true nature and potential to blossom.

The Taoist Internal Arts

The techniques of Taoist self-development are collectively known as the internal arts. They are considered arts because, although a precise theory underlies them, their actual practice is a creative process: since each person's condition is unique, their path is also unique. They are considered internal because they relate to your own being – both physically and at the level of your mind and emotions.

The techniques involve working with the internal processes and structures of the body and mind. This differentiates them from external practices such as physical exercise and gymnastics, which work only with the external physical structures of the body. The Chinese term for the internal arts is nei jia. Nei, meaning internal, leads to another term, nei gung, which means "internal work" and represents the methods that underlie all the internal arts. It is a more

Below A Taoist adept engaged in internal self-development practice. These arts lead the practitioner into an ever-deepening journey into their own nature, with complete freedom as the goal.

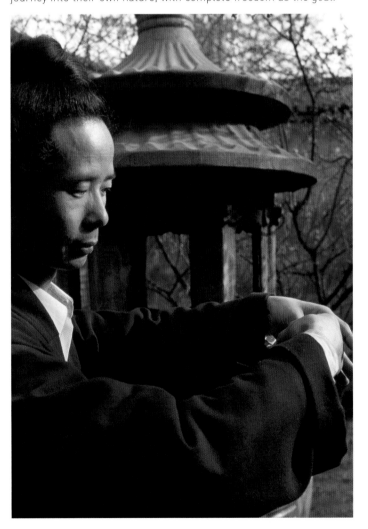

precise term than chi gung, as it specifically refers to the deeper Taoist self-development practices. The internal arts can be focused purely on upgrading health, or may include emotional, mental and spiritual development.

The Taoists found that the internal techniques could also be applied to the martial arts, which in ancient China were not sports or pastimes, but arose from a real need for self-defence in lawless and dangerous times. The nei gung techniques that give greater health, relaxation, clarity of mind and energy can also be used to generate incredible power. Accomplished practitioners of the "internal martial arts" are able to move and react in a way that could easily overcome most attackers, especially those using "external" techniques. Apart from their superiority as martial arts, what makes these practices so beneficial is that they inherently involve self-development practice. In fact, this is why they work so well as martial arts.

WU WEI

The highest level of these arts is the state of wu wei, which can be translated as "non-doing" or "empty action". Wu wei is a key principle in Taoism, as it implies a state of oneness with the Tao, "going with the flow" of the universe with no sense of imposing your own concepts or wishes on what is happening. In this state you act with total appropriateness to every situation, whether you are defending your life or making a cup of tea. There is no need for analytical thought: you respond naturally and effortlessly. In small ways we all experience this. For instance, if you accidentally touch something hot you pull your hand away without a moment's thought or hesitation. In that instant, you are in a state of wu wei. Athletes call this being "in the zone", where everything is perfect and effortless – like a surfer yielding to the flow of a wave. Applying the principle to all life's complex activities is the true challenge. Paradoxically, it is through deliberate training methods and long practice that you aim to transcend those very methods and truly enter wu wei.

A phrase in the t'ai chi classics, "Forget yourself and follow the Other", is a statement of the principle of wu wei. The "Other" is the Tao, the natural flow of events within

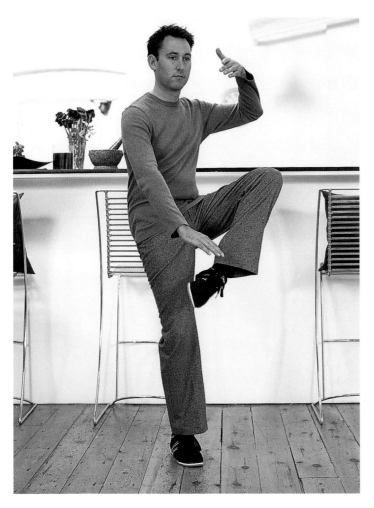

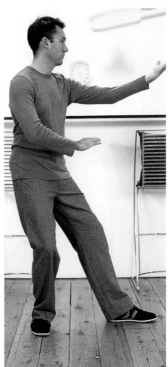

Below A posture from the single palm change of ba gua zhang. Studying the other two Taoist internal martial arts of ba gua and hsing-i can shed new light on one's experience of t'ai chi.

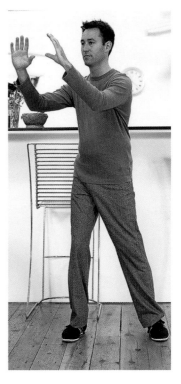

Below "Gods playing in the clouds" is a chi gung system containing all the Taoist nei gung principles. As these skills develop, they are incorporated into one's t'ai chi practice.

Above The various postures of the Wu style t'ai chi long form open different parts of the body and promote specific energy flows. Every posture is also a martial technique.

which you find yourself. Letting go of your ideas about what should happen, or what you would like to happen, and going with the flow, implies that you are not bound by your own ideas and concepts – in other words you are truly soong.

INTERNAL MARTIAL ARTS

There are three Taoist internal martial arts, all sharing the same Taoist nei gung foundations, but differing in the way they utilize these principles and methods. The most widely known, especially in the West, is t'ai chi chuan ("supreme ultimate fist"). Less well known are the arts of hsing-i chuan ("mind-form fist") and ba gua zhang ("eight trigram palm"). T'ai chi chuan is the easiest of the three to learn – typically it is said that everybody can learn t'ai chi but fewer can learn hsing-i and fewer still ba gua.

T'ai chi is based on and embodies yin/yang theory – it is primarily concerned with an unceasing flow from yin to yang and back again, both physically and in the energy and mind. It is essentially yin in nature (especially the Wu style, which is featured in this book) and is a superb method of relaxation and stress relief. This may account for its current popularity in the West. The stressed-out, yang nature of modern life requires a yin antidote, and t'ai chi is perfect. It is also an excellent method of healing the body, particularly

for correcting back, neck and joint problems – common results of stressful office work and sedentary lifestyles.

Hsing-i is based on Five Element theory, both the Generating (sheng) Cycle and the Controlling (ko) Cycle, in which each element or phase of energy has its antagonistic element: for example, Wood is "cut" by Metal. Hsing-i is strongly yang in nature, and its martial nature is very visible. It is externally simpler than t'ai chi, but as advanced internally, and is a useful art for those who are excessively yin or lack self-esteem, as it develops and sharpens the will and the ego. It is not ideal for those who are excessively yang; such people need a more yin practice such as t'ai chi.

Ba gua is based on the I Ching, and is the only purely Taoist internal art, as it has no elements of external martial forms within it. It is based on the very ancient Taoist circle walking meditation, and it embodies change – the constant flux of energies in the universe – as its core principle. As such it has a continuously moving, flowing and changing quality. It is generally considered to be the most sophisticated of the Taoist internal arts, and consequently the most difficult to master.

All these arts involve the cultivation of the energy centre in the abdomen known as the lower tantien ("elixir field") – pronounced "dandien". The lower tantien, usually referred to simply as the tantien, is the central point of all the body's chi energy, and therefore its cultivation is immensely beneficial for increasing martial power, attaining robust health, longevity and the energy needed to be fully active.

Chinese Medicine

Perhaps the most widely known of all the Taoist arts and sciences is Chinese medicine. Chinese medicine takes a typically Taoist view: that to achieve health and heal illness a holistic view of the patient is needed. This means taking not only their physical state and circumstances into account, but also their mental and emotional state: the idea that the two cannot really be separated is central to Chinese medicine.

A person's lifestyle choices and physical health are a reflection of their mental and emotional state, and vice versa; illness is seen as a result of imbalance in chi energy, with different types of imbalance resulting in different illnesses. Even infectious diseases are deemed to be a result of the body's lack of protective energy, or wei chi, which has allowed "invasion" by a pathogen. In a healthy, energetically balanced individual, the wei chi is strong and prevents pathogens from entering and causing illness.

Chinese doctors were traditionally paid a regular fee to maintain the health of their patients; if a patient fell ill the doctor would not be paid until they had restored the patient's health. So the paradigm of focusing on health rather than sickness was taken very literally indeed.

THE THREE TREASURES

Chinese medical theory is based on the concept of the three treasures, jing, chi and shen. Jing can be translated as "essence", chi as "energy" and shen as "spirit". Jing represents core energy – both the essential energy you were born with and that needed to maintain life. "Pre-birth" jing

Below Chinese herbalists measure out the components of a formula. Certain combinations of herbs will benefit specific health conditions. Herbs are particularly good for nourishing chi and blood.

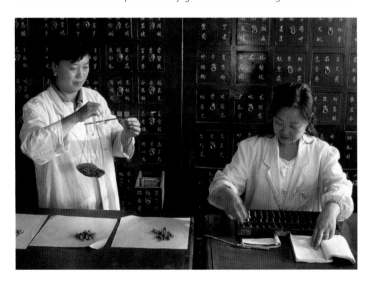

is your genetic inheritance, and determines your overall constitution and lifespan. As you age, it is slowly used up, and this is seen as the cause of ageing. When your pre-birth jing is exhausted, so is your life. In general, the amount of pre-birth jing is fixed at birth and cannot be added to (although there are advanced Taoist longevity practices that can enhance it). "Post-birth" jing is created from the food you eat and the air you breathe, as well as energy absorbed from your surroundings, such as sunlight, the cosmos or trees. If your post-birth jing is strong you feel that your core energy is good; if not, you feel drained. When you expend too much energy you temporarily exhaust your post-birth jing; if you do not rest and restore it, you start tapping into your irreplaceable pre-birth jing. This can cause premature ageing and permanent "burn-out". Practising t'ai chi can, over time, increase your store of post-birth jing, thus boosting your core energy reserves.

Chi is the active energy flowing through the body, and can be said to be produced from jing. If jing is the water, chi is the steam. It flows through specific channels in your body, sometimes called meridians, and takes many forms. It can be seen as your available energy, both for internal processes such as digestion and for external activity. The flow of chi varies according to the time, the seasons and even the movement of the stars and planets. Ill health occurs when the flow is disrupted by being blocked, scattered or even reversed. Since the physical body relies on healthy chi flow to sustain its structures and processes, ill health will result when imbalance occurs. The physical structures of the body are seen both as the result of, and the conduit for, chi flows. Physical injury can block the flow of chi, and vice versa: blocked or abnormal chi flow can result in physical abnormalities, such as skin disorders.

The third treasure, and the most subtle, is shen. This refers to mental/emotional aspects, as well as even more subtle "spiritual" levels. The state of a person's shen is said to be visible in their eyes, just as in the Western saying, "The eyes are the windows of the soul." A weak shen may result in depression, timidity or fearfulness. A disturbed shen would manifest as neurosis, or even mania and psychosis.

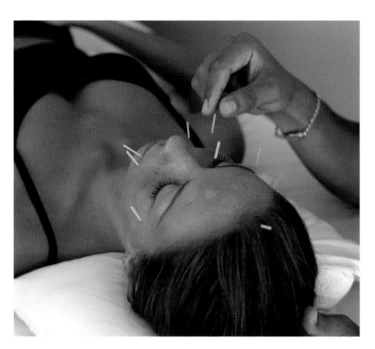

Left Acupuncture can be used to treat a variety of conditions, ranging from minor to life-threatening illnesses, and also for cosmetic rejuvenation treatments, such as the facial acupuncture session shown here.

While its exact nature is complex, it can be said to relate above all to the heart. If the shen is disturbed it will affect the state of a person's chi, while an imbalance of chi will eventually affect the shen, so they are mutually dependent. Since jing and chi are also mutually dependent, Chinese medicine always takes all three treasures into account when diagnosing and treating illness.

DIAGNOSIS

Practitioners diagnose a patient on the basis of many observations. One primary method is the taking of pulses on each wrist, with specific positions relating to specific organs of the body. The pulses are assessed on the basis of their speed and regularity and their quality: terms such as "empty", "choppy", "wiry" and "slippery" are used to denote its energetic quality. Taking the pulses can be an extremely powerful diagnostic tool, and is an art in itself. Observation of the patient's tongue will also yield key information about the state of the internal organs, with specific areas of the tongue relating to certain organs and functions of the body. In many ways, tongue diagnosis is less subjective. The results of the two are compared to form a fuller picture.

Observation of the patient's physical state and the way they move, talk and behave are also key diagnostic tools, with specific signs and attributes providing clues to underlying conditions. The practitioner will then ask a series of questions – some very similar to those a Western physician would ask, others very different, such as what kind of emotions the patient feels. A picture is thus built up of the physical, energetic and mental/emotional state of the patient in terms of Chinese medical theory (which uses several paradigms to categorize symptoms), and like a detective assembling seemingly separate pieces of evidence, the practitioner can then form a diagnosis and treatment plan.

The internal organs of the body play a major part in treatment, and the main channels or meridians each relate to an organ. The organs are divided into yin or zang organs, and yang or fu organs. Zang and fu are then paired according to the elements they represent and embody. The zang organs are seen to be of primary importance, and are also associated with certain emotions, as well as sounds, tastes, colours, smells and so on.

TREATMENT

Some treatments intervene with the patient's chi from the outside. Acupuncture uses very fine needles to access and correct the flow of chi within the channels at specific points, known as "cavities". A powerful herb – moxa, or mugwort – is sometimes burned above or on an acupuncture point, or even on the end of a needle, to move and tonify the chi: this is called "moxibustion". Another method of treatment is "cupping", where glass or bamboo jars are briefly heated and then placed on the body, creating a vacuum as the air within them cools. Chinese herbal medicine works from inside the body to transform the patterns of chi flow, especially with regard to the organs, or zang-fu. Herbs take longer to act but generally do so on a deep level. The practice of tui na, often called Chinese massage, is used as a form of body therapy to release bindings and blockages in the tissues, while simultaneously working with the acupuncture channels to effect change on a deeper level.

Traditionally a Chinese physician not only treats a patient but also offers them lifestyle advice, including dietary advice, and instructs them in chi gung techniques for self-healing. In many cases this includes a recommendation to take up t'ai chi as a way of maintaining robust health, as it utilizes the core principles of Chinese medicine, and represents a powerful method of self-treatment.

Below Acupuncture needles and mugwort herb, burned in stick form or on the ends of needles to warm cold and deficient areas.

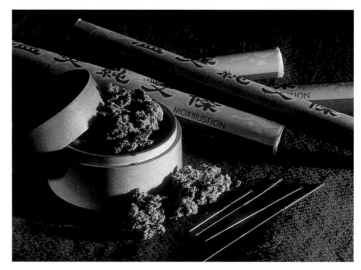

Chi Gung and Nei Gung

A person's chi energy can be stronger or weaker depending on their state of health – physical, mental and emotional – and also on their basic constitution. While Chinese medicine seeks to redress any imbalances in the flow of chi within a patient, chi gung ("energy work") practice enables a person to remove blockages in their own chi and actually increase their available energy, both immediately and in the long term.

Chi gung is a generic term for all types of Chinese energetic self-development work, and the practices it describes vary enormously in both underlying theory and application. The term is becoming increasingly familiar in the West, though Chinese energetic practices are latecomers compared to Indian yoga techniques, which established a foothold decades earlier. Chi gung is usually understood to imply methods that use a series of movements involving breathing work. In many ways this is not inaccurate, but as chi gung becomes increasingly popular in the West, the differences between the systems in existence will also become more evident. In fact, there are several chi gung traditions in China: medical, martial, Buddhist, Confucian and Taoist. Each has a distinct character and approach, reflecting its origins. Though some aspects of the systems overlap, others differ widely.

Below A core principle in t'ai chi is to integrate the inner with the outer, and internal practice with the external elements.

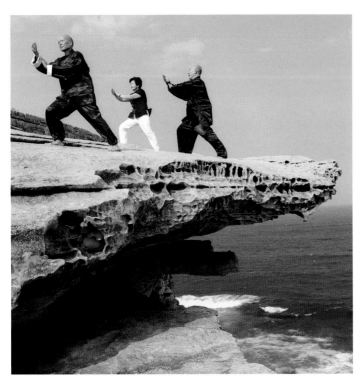

INSIDE AND OUTSIDE

The term nei gung, particularly Taoist nei gung, is much more specific. What most distinguishes nei gung from other chi gung practices is the difference between nei – the internal – and wei – the external. While nei gung methods work from the inside (the core of the body) to the outside, the opposite is true of other chi gung methods. Like acupuncture, which by accessing relatively superficial energetic channels seeks to have an effect on the organs and deeper systems of the body, chi gung often uses external movements and breathing techniques to do this. Chi gung also works one aspect of the body's energetic systems at a time, often building these techniques into a sequential set of movements.

Within each chi gung tradition there are many techniques, and some systems are highly effective, especially at removing chi stagnation, while others are not. The value of any chi gung system lies in how well it works in relation to the time and effort required from the practitioner. Many chi gung practices are easier to learn and apply than the more advanced nei gung methods. However, the potential benefits of nei gung practice are substantially greater than those available from more external chi gung practices.

An important principle of nei gung is that whatever you do at the deeper levels of your being has a great effect on all the more superficial levels: one unit of time and effort at a deep level can have ten units of effect on the shallower levels. Conversely, it takes ten units of time and effort at the shallower levels to achieve one unit of effect at the deeper levels. Therefore, according to nei gung theory, it is more useful to work directly at the deeper levels of your body and energy from the start. This is, of course, harder to achieve as the deeper levels are more "hidden", but it can be done, with a little application, by almost anybody.

One of the more immediate advantages of nei gung practice is that it allows for the release of deep tensions and blockages in the physical body, allowing the healing of even long-standing spinal and joint problems and also an improvement in the functioning of the internal organs. These benefits might never be attained with external chi

Right A movement from "dragon and tiger" chi gung. Practising chi gung alongside t'ai chi can greatly enhance a person's ability to work with chi energy.

Below Many of the nei gung components of t'ai chi are more easily developed separately, before being integrated into one's t'ai chi practice.

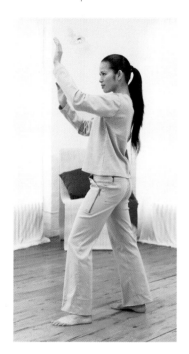

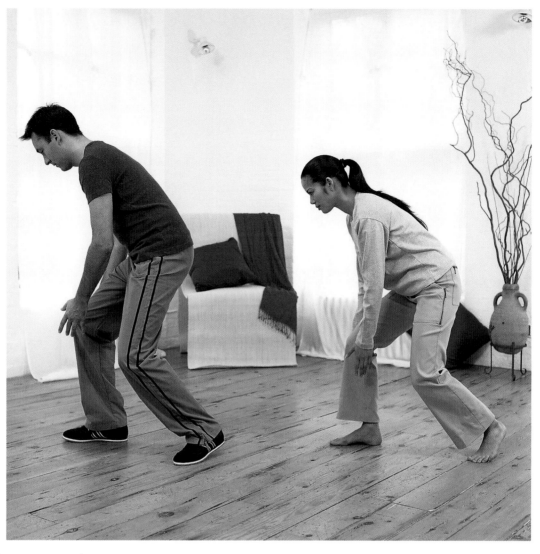

gung systems, many of which (though not all) are concerned mainly with developing chi – increasing the amount of power in the system. This is fine in a healthy, balanced body, but almost everybody has energetic (and physical) blockages that do not need to be "powered up", but instead need to be released. For most people the problem is not of a fundamental lack of energy, but of blockages in their energy flow, and this can manifest as a lack of available energy for a particular part of the body, or even overall. In a blocked water pipe, you would not want simply to increase the pressure, or the pipe might burst. Instead you would want to dissolve away the blockage to allow normal flow to resume. Nei gung methods seek first to release energetic blockages and correct physical misalignments before developing natural energetic capacity. Nei gung embodies the Taoist principle of naturalness – of regaining a natural healthy state that is inherently vibrant and powerful.

NEI GUNG TECHNIQUES

The techniques can be subdivided into several categories. They include opening and closing ("pulsing") of all the joints and tissues; spiralling of all the tissues; working with the energy flows of the deepest channels; dissolving blockages in all the energetic bodies; working with the energy of the spine and spinal cord; and breathing techniques (nei gung does not rely on breathing to move the chi – the mind is used directly – but breathing may be used where appropriate). These are just a few of the Taoist nei gung techniques. Although they are usually learned singly, once mastered they are performed simultaneously. Thus nei gung practice may involve just one simple movement, within which all the nei gung methods are being applied at the same time. This creates a synergy that dramatically increases the effectiveness of the practice – it becomes more than just the sum of its parts.

NEI GUNG AND T'AI CHI

When performed correctly, t'ai chi is a nei gung practice – and this is also true of hsing-i and ba gua. After you have learned the t'ai chi form – the sequence of external movements – you will want to start introducing nei gung principles and components into your practice, one at a time. As you do this your form may change little on the outside, at least to the casual observer, but your personal experience of practising t'ai chi will change and evolve dramatically. Ultimately, a dedicated t'ai chi practitioner seeks to incorporate all the nei gung methods into their form, making it a very powerful and sophisticated nei gung practice. This is where the deeper benefits of t'ai chi are to be found, and where it truly becomes an internal art.

The Origins and Development of T'ai Chi

The exact origins of t'ai chi chuan are the subject of endless controversy, as there is no way of verifying which of the many theories about it are true. One thing is certain: t'ai chi first appeared in the Chen village in China at some time during the 16th century. Another certainty is that from the outset it had Taoist influence. The following story may or may not be true – but it is very likely.

A master named Wang Tsung Yueh arrived at the Chen village and visited the local inn. Over the course of an evening, the subject of martial arts was discussed – this was at a time when such skills were essential for survival in the face of organized banditry. The locals (all of the same clan) were very proud of their external Shaolin style martial art called pao twi or "cannon fist". Wang was unimpressed and told them so in no uncertain terms. Deeply insulted, the villagers attacked Wang, but he beat off his multiple attackers in a way they had never seen before. Amazed and humbled, they begged Wang to teach them his art. Wang agreed, but as he did not have time to teach them his complete system, he modified their existing external martial art to include Taoist nei gung methods – making it fully "internal". This new art – Chen style t'ai chi – continued to develop, and today is one of the three main styles of t'ai chi.

Where Wang Tsung Yueh learned his art will probably never be known. A well-known legend is that t'ai chi or its antecedent was created by the Taoist "Immortal" Chang San Feng after he watched a snake and a crane fighting. Whatever the truth, the involvement of Taoist sages in the creation and development of the internal martial arts can be taken for granted, as they all contain fundamental Taoist nei gung practices.

T'AI CHI EVOLVES

In the 19th century a master named Yang Lu Chan (1799–1872) further developed the art and spread t'ai chi beyond the Chen village. As a young man he had been tutored by the Chen clan – no mean feat, as t'ai chi was at the time their secret weapon, unique to the clan. Yang travelled all over China and accepted all challenges, never losing once, and never seriously injuring his opponents, no matter how violent. He became known as "Yang the

Below The art of t'ai chi, and the Taoist wisdom it embodies, has spread outwards from its origins in remote parts of China, to be practised by millions of people throughout the world today.

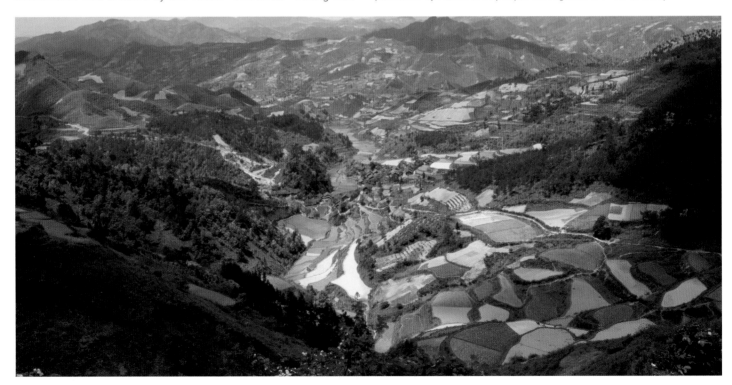

Right A female practitioner of t'ai chi straight sword. T'ai chi weapons also include the sabre, spear and wooden staff. Weapons practice can help develop strength, balance and spiralling energy.

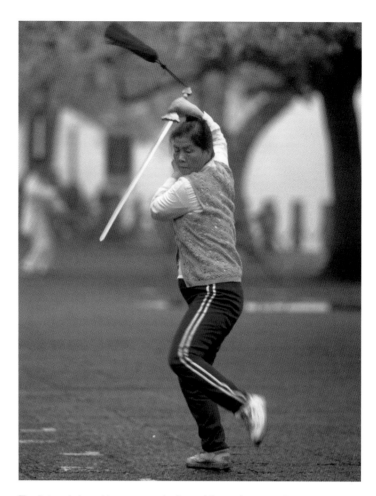

Invincible". He was accepted as the finest martial artist in all China, and taught the Emperor's bodyguards. He also accepted other students, one of whom was Wu Yu Hsiang, whose "small frame" style of t'ai chi later became known as the Hao style. While a valid style of t'ai chi, Hao style is not considered to be one of the main styles, and neither is the Sun style of Sun Lu Tang, which is a fusion of all three of the Taoist internal martial arts.

Yang style flourished, and was known as Yang Family style as it was mainly passed from father to son: Yang Lu Chan passed it to his son Yang Pan Hou, who in turn passed it to his son Yang Chen Fu. It changed somewhat with Yang Chen Fu, losing some of its highly martial emphasis, and this is known as "new" Yang style. The changes were largely to do with the change in attitudes to the traditional martial arts in China after the Boxer Rebellion in 1900. This catastrophic event was a desperate attempt by the Emperor to expel foreign powers from Beijing, using martial artists ("boxers") from all over China. The foreign forces used machine guns and the result was carnage, and a total rout of the boxers. China was divided among the victors, and Chinese martial arts never regained their almost mythical status in the face of the stark reality of modern firearms. Yang style t'ai chi, however, survived, and continues to flourish.

WU STYLE T'AI CHI

Yang Lu Chan's top student, Chuan You, was adept at the most advanced, transformational aspect of t'ai chi energy work, and developed his art based on these principles. He later taught his son, Wu Jien Chuan (1870–1942), who also studied with Yang Pan Hou (Yang Lu Chan's son). Wu Jien Chuan taught with the Yang family in Beijing and he and Yang Chen Fu often demonstrated their t'ai chi side by side. Wu Jien Chuan, being 20 years the senior of the two, also helped Yang Chen Fu develop his skills.

Partly because of the transformational energy work that had been passed on to him by his father, and partly because he was also a Taoist spiritual practitioner, Wu Jien Chuan's interests lay increasingly in the inner aspects of t'ai chi, especially its potential for healing and meditation. This was in no way incompatible with the martial aspect, as the power, sensitivity and subtlety that can be accessed at the deeper levels of being inherently allow for superior martial ability. Wu consequently evolved his t'ai chi style to operate at the deepest levels, seeking to make its movements and energy flows originate from the practitioner's core. This was in keeping with Taoist nei gung principles of accessing the deepest levels possible at every stage. It could be said that Wu Jien Chuan was attempting to take t'ai chi closer to its

Taoist origins. He succeeded, as his style contains techniques that relate directly to Taoist nei gung, some of which are not so heavily emphasized in the other styles, or are entirely absent. The result was a "small frame" style of t'ai chi, where the external movements are not as pronounced but the internal movements are in fact larger.

LINEAGE

Wu taught openly, and as a result Wu style t'ai chi is widely known in China, and is arguably more popular than the Yang style in parts of southern China. The secretive days of the Chen village had passed and the art could be spread for the benefit of many. However, its deeper aspects and techniques would always be reserved for those worthy of the knowledge and capable of absorbing and understanding it. Thus the principle of lineage was, and still is, upheld.

The complete art was passed only to those few students whom the master accepted as formal disciples. The main reason for this was and is the importance of keeping the knowledge alive and intact, ensuring it is not "watered down", confused or lost. It is also a guarantee of quality – if you are training with a lineage master you know that what is being passed to you is authentic and effective. It is not always possible to train with such a teacher, but the closer your teacher is to a genuine lineage, the greater the likelihood that you will be well trained. T'ai chi will inevitably evolve in the future, but in the hands of creative and talented masters the knowledge and skill that has been passed down will provide the foundations for the art as it develops.

The Different Styles of Tai Chi

Although there are differences between the various styles of t'ai chi, key similarities are shared by all the authentic styles. It is these similarities that distinguish t'ai chi from other martial, movement and energetic arts, and mark the authenticity of a t'ai chi style. If a style is lacking any of the core principles it cannot truly be said to be t'ai chi, though it might look like it: it will be only, as the Chinese say, "waving your arms in the air".

While many t'ai chi practitioners like to claim that their style is the "real thing", all genuine practitioners are essentially practising the same art, only with differences in emphasis. Just as the members of a family have different characters, interests and dispositions, so the various styles of t'ai chi have different emphases and approaches. The goal of all authentic t'ai chi is the same: the state of wu wei and the merging with the Ultimate, or t'ai chi. All styles also share the goals of superior personal health and energy, longevity, mental stillness and clarity, and effective self-defence.

Where the main styles differ is in their use of some of these principles, their approach to fighting techniques and, above all, in their approach to energetic development. A casual observer watching the three main styles being performed would be most likely to notice the following differences, which hint at quite dramatic differences in terms of the internal work of the following three styles.

Below Wu style posture "fan through the back". In this style this posture is a meditation point. The body is opened evenly to allow for a fuller sense of "letting go" from one's centre.

Below In the Wu style of t'ai chi the spine is allowed to lean on certain moves, while remaining straight along its length. Yang style t'ai chi adopts a more upright posture at all times.

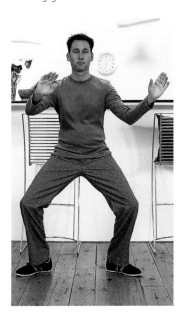
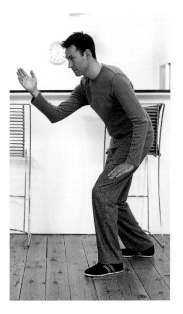

DIFFERENCES IN THE CHEN, YANG AND WU STYLES

Chen style has highly visible spiralling motions, both in the arms and the body as a whole. It is quite "gymnastic", involving jumps and leaps. The pace changes from very slow to very rapid. It employs visible shaking, vibrating moves when issuing energy, as well as stamping foot movements. It looks a little like Shaolin-type kung fu, which is apt, given its closeness to t'ai chi's "ancestor", pao twi.

Yang style appears much smoother than Chen style, without the acrobatic leaps and twists. Spiralling motions are hard to see as they are internal, and it usually maintains an even pace. It does not use the overt shaking and stamping movements of the Chen style. It typifies the popular image of t'ai chi – smooth, slow and peaceful.

Wu style appears to use much smaller movements than the Yang style, with both the stance and the arm positions less extended. It also appears to be "higher", as the practitioner may not bend the legs so much. Any spiralling motions are all but invisible in the Wu style. The practitioner appears to be doing less, and it may appear more "casual" than the Yang style. In certain postures the spine leans forward, whereas in Yang style it is nearly always vertical.

CHEN STYLE

The Chen style was originally used on the battlefield by armoured warriors wielding weapons. This shaped its form considerably, for instance, its gymnastic quality may be a result of the need to move quickly while encumbered by armour. Probably the most obvious difference between the Chen and later styles is in the visible use of chan ssu jin, or "silk-reeling" energy. The name refers to the way silk is drawn from a cocoon: it must be done with a smooth twisting action, or the threads will break. Chi moves in a spiral motion; to maximize the flow of chi in yourself you therefore need to use spiralling motions in the body. This is one of the key principles of t'ai chi, and in the Chen style it is highly visible as an external coiling movement. Energetically, Chen style seeks to develop "hard" or yang energy. This should not be confused with tensing the muscles as all styles of t'ai chi involve muscular relaxation.

Right The posture ji or "push" in the Yang style. Note the wider stance and position of the arms.

Far right Ji in the Wu style. Note the narrower stance and the hands located on the centreline.

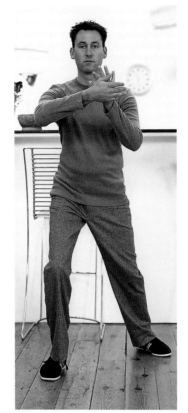 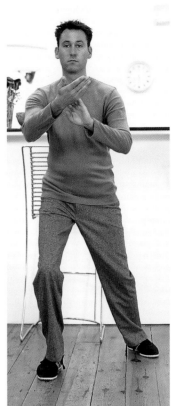

YANG STYLE

T'ai chi was dramatically changed by Yang Lu Chan. Yang's was an age of firearms: armoured warriors became an anachronism, and the reasons for many of the Chen style's characteristics no longer existed. The spiralling elbow of Chen style became more dropped and relaxed; there were no jumps and leaps; stances were weighted 100 per cent on one leg and 0 per cent on the other. Chan ssu jin was achieved by spiralling the tissues of the limbs rather than the limbs as a whole; this became known as "pulling silk" because the emphasis was on directly drawing energy from and into the spine and lower tantien (the body's energy centre). Overall, the energetic work became more internalized, relying less on external motions and more on subtle motions within the body. Many Yang style masters went "smaller" in their form through the course of their lives. The energetic emphasis shifted from the development of hard, yang energy to soft, yin energy, eventually fusing the two. The Yang style works primarily on the external energy field of the body, which is useful for martial projection of energy, called fa jin, or "issuing power".

WU STYLE

The trend of internalization of t'ai chi methods continued with the Wu style, which incorporates Taoist meditation methods and a wider range of nei gung techniques. While spiralling actions are just visible in the Yang style, they are practically invisible in the Wu style, as they are done deep within the tissues. The Yang style opens up the outside of the body first, using large and extended postures, and later seeks to open the inside of the body. The Wu style, does the opposite, using smaller postures to access the inside of the body first, then letting those releases spread to the outside. This is the principle of "small on the outside, large on the inside": small external movements allow for larger internal movements, while large external movements usually allow only small internal movements.

While in the Yang style the progression is from external to internal, the Wu style starts with the internal. It works mainly with the deep side channels of the body, as it is more concerned with moving and transforming energy within the body than outside it. In the Wu style, described as "small frame", the hand positions relate to activating the deep channels of the body, rather than the external field. The elbows point down, creating a greater release in the deep side channels and greater internal pressures.

The Wu style places major emphasis on transforming energy rather than only moving it. This can make it superior for healing damage to the body's tissues and systems,

which need to be transformed and repaired and not just strengthened. Certain postures in the Wu style are designed to open and release the central energy channel – a Taoist meditation technique that is not found in other styles of t'ai chi. In its movements, Wu style t'ai chi generally uses more spheres, while the Yang style uses mainly circles. In Wu style the wrist pulse is often touched to lead into awareness of the internal organs. A very visible difference is the leaning forward on the bending moves in Wu style. This was introduced to allow a more natural action while maintaining an internally straight spine along the angle of lean. Some moves in Wu style use 45° angles in the hands rather than the flat planes found in the Yang style. Energetically, the Wu style seeks to develop soft, yin energy first and then to find hard, yang energy from the emptiness of the soft; this allows for a greater release of tension and healing from the start, but the Wu style is also somewhat harder to master than the opposite approach.

CHOOSING A STYLE

It would be true to say that the Wu style places emphasis on healing and meditation, while Yang style emphasizes the development of energetic power, but it is important to remember that the Wu style is an evolution of the Yang style, and not a radically different art. The postures and form sequence are largely the same, although their execution can differ. The true destination of t'ai chi is the same whatever the style, and the route you take depends on your nature and interests. Those who are yin by nature may find a yang approach works for them, and may be drawn to the Yang style. If you are more yang, or have an interest in meditation, you may be drawn to the yin approach of the Wu style.

Hsing-i and Ba Gua

Although all three Taoist internal martial arts share the underpinnings of Taoist nei gung methods, they appear quite different to the observer, and can feel quite different to the practitioner. This is because they utilize nei gung components in differing ways, each with a distinct approach and emphasis. Each has its own philosophical and spiritual approach, all with the same goal but taking different paths to reach it.

HSING-I CHUAN – MIND-FORM FIST

T'ai chi is based on yin/yang theory, and has an overall yin nature. Hsing-i is the opposite: both its energetic quality and its mental approach are very yang in nature. While t'ai chi has a yielding mental attitude, never meeting force with force but instead flowing around it and influencing it with the minimum of effort, hsing-i is aggressive, preferring to meet an opponent head-on and overwhelm them by greater force, applied correctly. Hsing-i is about imposing your will on your opponent. The "i" in hsing-i means "intent": you decide what you want to do, and do it; if your opponent is in the way, you simply crash through them. Hsing-i attacks continuously – even when you are retreating you continue to strike at your opponent. Yang energy is present constantly, never yielding.

Hsing-i tends to move in straight lines, even when changing direction: it zig-zags. This is visibly different from the circular movements of t'ai chi and ba gua. It looks like an internal form of karate – linear and aggressive – but it differs in that it uses no muscular tension or anger (emotional tension). Its power comes from its nei gung, just like t'ai chi and ba gua. Unlike t'ai chi, however, it is almost always performed at high speed, with all movement originating in the fist or hand, as opposed to the tantien as in t'ai chi.

According to legend, hsing-i was created by Yue Fei, reputedly the greatest general in Chinese history. This hints at its aggressive, no-nonsense militaristic quality as a fighting art. In a sense, it is simpler than t'ai chi or ba gua, as it uses a minimum of techniques. Being based on Five Element theory, it possesses five main techniques: pi chuan or "splitting fist", which is Metal; tsuan chuan or "drilling fist", which is Water; beng chuan or "crushing fist", which is Wood; pao chuan or "pounding fist", which is Fire; and heng chuan or "crossing fist", which is Earth. Each develops the energy of its element within the practitioner and will benefit the corresponding organs: "splitting fist", for example, benefits the lungs, which are Metal in nature. In hsing-i fighting, these elemental techniques are used to defeat the opponent's techniques according to the ko (controlling) cycle

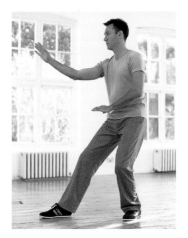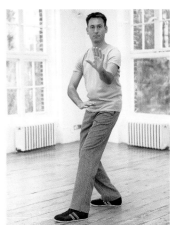

Above The pi chuan "splitting fist" technique of hsing-i is shown on the left, and the circle walking posture of ba gua on the right.

of the Five Elements; for instance, "splitting fist" (Metal) tends to overcome "pounding fist", which is Wood. The five main techniques can be linked and developed in what are known as animal forms.

Hsing-i is extremely effective as a martial art, placing its main emphasis on the development of internal power to deliver devastating strikes to an opponent. This power is mainly developed through the use of a standing posture called san ti. This is the "splitting fist" technique frozen in time, and is therefore Metal in quality. Over time, san ti develops the internal energy of the practitioner and also the mental focus, developing an iron will ("i"). This can then direct the body to produce a form ("hsing") that is infused with internal energy. Hsing-i does not appeal to the average person – it is overtly martial and its training methods are fairly arduous – but in the dedicated practitioner it can create a very strong mind and body. It is said of hsing-i that "It's not pretty, but it works."

BA GUA ZHANG – EIGHT TRIGRAM PALM

With a distinctly different quality and methodology to hsing-i and t'ai chi, the art of ba gua zhang surfaced in Beijing in 1852 with a master called Tung Hai Chuan. Tung never fully explained where he had learned ba gua zhang, but claimed

T'AI CHI IN CONTEXT

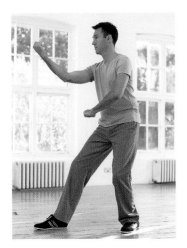 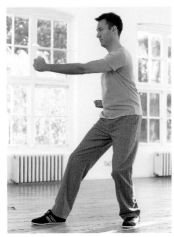

Above Hsing-i: on the left is tsuan chuan "drilling fist" – the Water element. Right is beng chuan "crushing fist" – the Wood element.

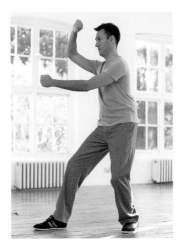 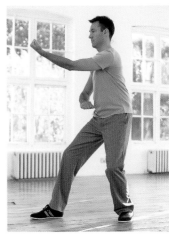

Above Hsing-i: on the left is pao chuan "pounding fist" – the Fire element. Right is heng chuan "crossing fist" – the Earth element.

that he learned it from an old Taoist sage in the mountains. It is certainly based on the ancient Taoist spiritual practice of circle walking meditation, but whether it was already developed as the complex internal martial art that Tung possessed will never be known. Tung Hai Chuan amazed the martial arts world of the time by beating all challengers with this strange and unique art. He became justly famous and passed the art on to a relatively small number of students, many of whose lineages survive to this day.

While t'ai chi has a yin quality, and hsing-i a yang quality, ba gua is concerned purely with change – it is not characteristically yin or yang, but flows between these poles with infinite permutations. Like hsing-i it is performed at speed, often lightning-fast. But unlike hsing-i it is extremely beautiful to watch, having a constantly flowing and coiling quality that does not resemble any other martial art – in fact it is quite unlike any other movement art.

This constancy of flow and change is perhaps the essential characteristic of ba gua – being the embodiment of change, it never hesitates and never stops. All the techniques, such as strikes and throws, are delivered on the move. While a t'ai chi practitioner takes a position, or "root", and executes a technique before changing position, a ba gua practitioner executes a technique as they are changing position. It is almost impossible to pin a good practitioner down – they are moving on at the very same moment that they are delivering a strike, throw or kick. This is made possible by the internal methodology of ba gua: there is a constant sense of coiling and uncoiling the body both internally and externally, and the practitioner is always "walking" – all movement originates in the feet. This allows for sudden changes of direction, allowing the practitioner to deal with multiple opponents simultaneously, flowing from one attacker to the next seamlessly and spontaneously.

The actual practice of ba gua zhang consists of "walking the circle". This opens the energy channels of the body and activates the upward and downward spiralling energy currents that pass through it. Then "single palm change" is practised, represented by chien, the trigram for heaven,

which is yang in nature. After this, practitioners develop the Double Palm Change, which is Earth and yin in nature. There are eight main or "mother" palm changes in ba gua, each symbolizing and embodying the energy of a trigram, with energetic qualities such as wind, thunder and fire. They are fast, complex changes of direction and energy that inherently contain martial techniques. Later these eight changes are developed into the 64 hexagrams of the I Ching, embodying all energetic change in the universe.

Higher levels of ba gua practice are linked to the principles of Taoist alchemy: transformation of the practitioner's internal energies, utilizing the energies of their surroundings and the cosmos. Crucial to this level of practice is the principle of spontaneity, merging with the Tao and allowing the flux of universal energies to determine the form that ba gua takes. Very few individuals reach this stage of accomplishment, but even at lower levels of skill, ba gua practice allows an understanding and acceptance of change to develop within, bringing about freedom from the rigid concepts that can limit creativity and human potential.

Below A detail from the second (double) palm change of ba gua, representing the trigram for Earth.

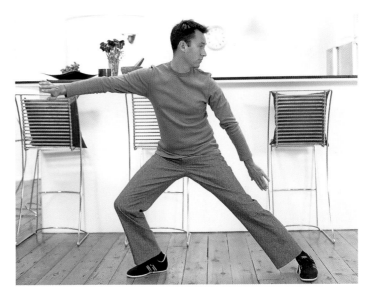

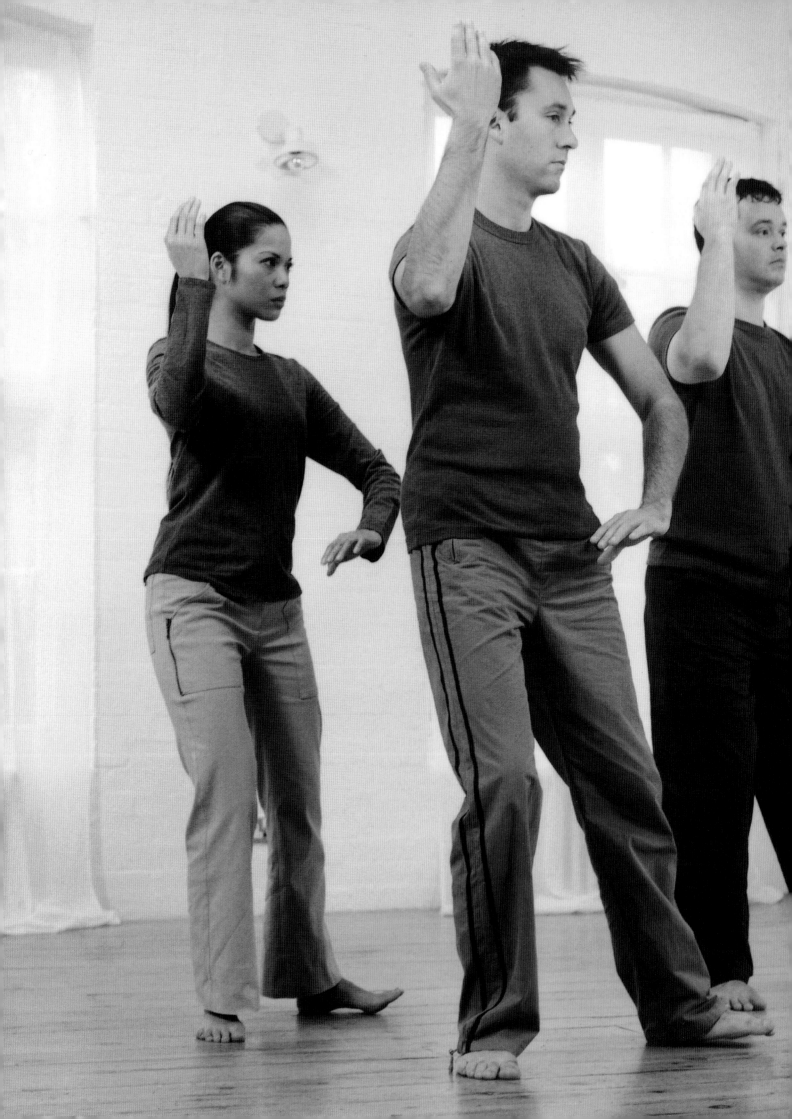

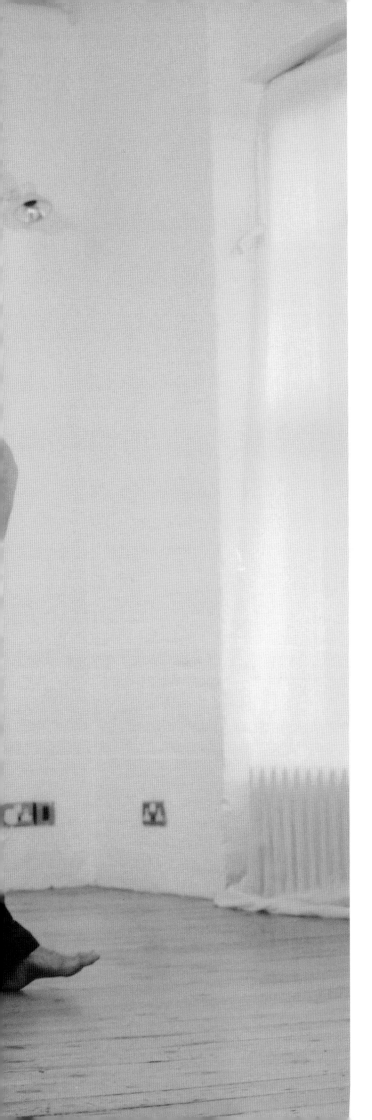

T'ai Chi for Mind and Body

The reasons for learning t'ai chi apply to everyone. As human beings we all face challenges to our physical, mental and emotional health. It is simply a question of what form these problems take and when in our lives they appear. Learning t'ai chi is about taking responsibility for your own well-being and taking action to improve it to secure a healthy and balanced future. This chapter looks first at what makes t'ai chi unique as a mind–body practice, then compares its main benefits with those of other exercise regimes. This is followed by an examination of the role of the body and mind connection in relation to t'ai chi practice, and a look at how this relates to meditation practice. The chapter ends with sections on the use of t'ai chi for healing back and neck problems, energizing, reducing stress and stilling the mind, and balancing the emotions.

A Unique Approach to Self-development

There are many possible approaches to self-development: some ancient, some modern, stemming from many different cultures and traditions. Many share common tenets, others take radically different views of what self-development means and how we should go about it. They can be broadly divided into those that work primarily with the body, primarily with energy and primarily with the mind.

Most self-development practices take one of these three approaches, usually with the view that the level on which they are focusing is the "correct" one with which to work. This is not in itself wrong, as each aspect is indeed fundamental to human existence. Therefore any practice that genuinely accesses one of these levels and leads to development and evolution is important and valid – no matter where or when it originated. However, from a Taoist viewpoint, working with only one or two aspects of a human being is not a complete practice of self-development.

THE THREE TREASURES
The Taoists consider the three treasures of jing, chi and shen to be inseparable. Jing relates to the physical body, chi to the energy of that body, and shen to the mind. Just as all three are treated together in Chinese medicine, so in Taoist self-development practice you work with all three at the

Below Working with body, energy and mind simultaneously is an inherent part of t'ai chi practice.

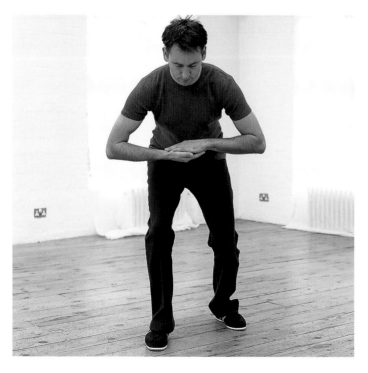

same time. To omit one or more from your practice means that you are working not with your complete being, only with certain aspects of yourself. This is important both to achieve health and also in relation to your spiritual development. You cannot achieve true physical health if your energy is not balanced, and your energy cannot be truly balanced unless your mind is also balanced. Most people are all too aware of how mental stress leads to physical illness – this is a perfect example of the interrelationship between mind and body. Therefore, even if your goal is purely to achieve robust and lasting physical health, you need to include the levels of energy and mind in your practice. Conversely, even if your goal is purely that of spiritual development, you need the support of a balanced body and energy to stabilize the mind: you need only observe someone who is ill or in chronic pain to see the effects of physical ill health on the mind.

Where certain systems of self-development fall short is in a partial approach: believing that one can effectively ignore any of these aspects of oneself and yet still achieve balanced progress. Put simply, this is not possible. The Taoists have always understood this, as have many other ancient traditions. Practices that seek to develop only the "spiritual" aspects of a person, without also developing physical and energetic aspects, rarely succeed, because the foundations of a relaxed and healthy body and energy are not present. Practices that seek to find the spiritual solely through physical and energetic work, thus neglecting the mind, also tend to fail. The answer lies in working with all three aspects simultaneously, and this is what t'ai chi does.

THE T'AI CHI APPROACH
The practice of t'ai chi involves working simultaneously with your physical body, your chi, and your mind. While there are many training methods connected to it that involve working on specific aspects, the actual practice of t'ai chi should always involve all three at the same time. This is not only to develop all three levels – arguably that could be achieved by working with them separately. When you work with body, energy and mind simultaneously, something unique occurs: the integration of all three. A synergy takes place that

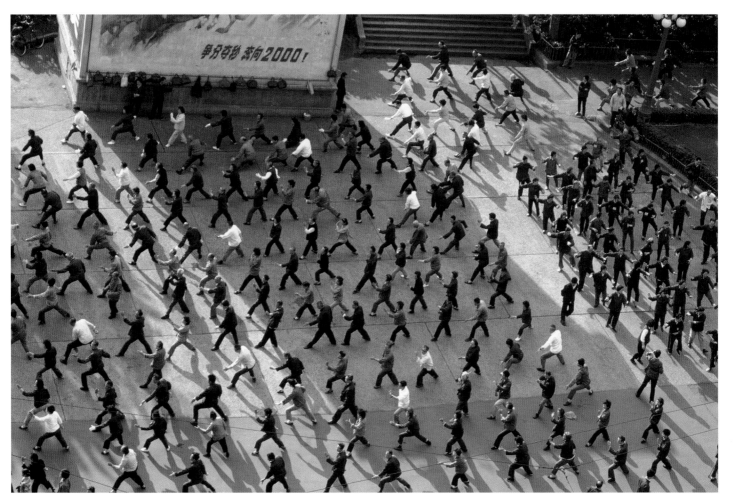

Above A typical scene in China, where huge groups practise t'ai chi amidst the noise and movement of city life, an illustration of how the art offers a means of achieving stillness within chaos.

dramatically increases the development of each of the levels. This is because in essence they are not separate; most people have just lost the natural integration within themselves and with the universe as a whole. By integrating your own existence, you begin integrating with all existence: this is spiritual development. However, even if you are not interested in spiritual development, but simply in obtaining better health and freedom from stress – and this is a perfectly valid motivation for wanting to learn t'ai chi – this integral method is invaluable in order to reap the greatest benefits from your time and effort.

T'ai chi involves movement and integration with the external world – the world outside of yourself, including other people – and therefore it can achieve something that purely inward-focused practices, such as many forms of sitting meditation, rarely do: the integration of your external (wei) and internal (nei) aspects. The practical effect of this is the ability to remain calm and centred even in the midst of stressful external circumstances, such as life in a big city or the work environment. In t'ai chi you learn to be inwardly and outwardly aware at the same time, and to retain stillness of mind within movement, both your own and that of the outside world. This is developed through solo practice of the t'ai chi form, and through two-person push hands practice.

T'ai chi is inherently a martial art, and so it also offers you an opportunity to identify and explore personal issues relating to the ego and your personal fears, in the context of a meditative practice. This can allow the release of tensions, including deep anger, that might otherwise be very elusive.

EVERYDAY LIFE
T'ai chi is relevant and timely in this increasingly hectic world. It provides a method of achieving inner and outer balance in the face of great pressures. It does not require you to abandon all worldly concerns and retreat to a mountain cave – in fact, that would not be considered a balanced approach to self-development as it would be excessively yin. Retreat may be an important part of your practice, whether for an hour or a month, but the art of t'ai chi evolved in the midst of life's swirling chaos, and as a practice it is quite comfortable there. It offers a means of achieving stillness within chaos, through patient daily practice. It is said, "One day's practice yields one day's results, one year's practice yields one year's results," meaning that by dedicating some time each day to t'ai chi practice, the benefits naturally grow. This has been compared to stacking one sheet of paper on top of another – each sheet seems to add almost nothing, but over time a tall pile of paper will be built up. Even half an hour of practice a day will yield excellent results over time. This is something that everybody can achieve, no matter how hectic their lifestyle, if they have a will to do it.

The Health Benefits of T'ai Chi

What distinguishes t'ai chi from other movement arts or forms of exercise is its use of the nei gung methods to release tensions within the body and to move and develop chi energy. This provides a host of benefits, many of which are not obtainable through ordinary exercise. T'ai chi is not simply a physical movement art: its movements and postures are the container within which you develop your chi.

Specific body alignments and movement patterns allow for the optimum flow of chi, and for releases to occur within the body, while avoiding chi "leaking" away. Because the physical movements are visible, they are the part that people recognize as "t'ai chi", but as your practice develops they will become only a part of a much greater experience. It is the internal work that distinguishes t'ai chi from other exercise systems and is responsible for its benefits.

T'AI CHI AND EXERCISE

Some exercise regimes adopt a "no pain, no gain" attitude that treats the body almost as an enemy to be vanquished, rather than as an integral part of yourself, and this can result in damage and accelerated ageing. In t'ai chi practice you always stay within your body's limits, not causing excessive wear, exhaustion or damage. The benefits of this approach can be seen in many practitioners in their 70s and 80s, who have physical flexibility, mental alertness and energy levels greater than most people half their age.

Below In t'ai chi one never locks any joints or induces any muscular tension, as this blocks the flow of chi in the body.

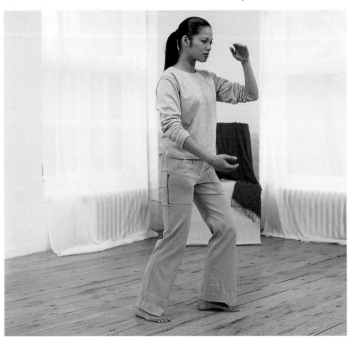

HEALTH

Fitness and health are not necessarily the same thing. You can become extremely fit, in terms of being able to run a marathon, and yet suffer ill health simultaneously, possibly as a result of the fitness training itself. Health is a state of balance, and you do not need extreme physical abilities in order to call yourself healthy.

The health benefits of t'ai chi can be divided into those relating to physical health, including energy levels, and those that relate to the mind and emotions. T'ai chi is known for restoring glowing health to the debilitated in a way that is hardly surpassed by any other system. Perhaps the most obvious feature of t'ai chi practice is that it involves constant gentle movement without strain. This allows for lubrication of the joints and regains space within them. A "drying up" and contraction of the joints occurs as you age, and t'ai chi can help to retain flexibility and general mobility

The pulsing (opening and closing) actions that take place within the joints and internal spaces of the body during t'ai chi practice cause body fluids, including cerebro-spinal fluid, to be smoothly distributed and circulated, nourishing all parts of the body, and allowing for the proper transportation of metabolic waste products, which can otherwise build up and cause disease. The constant bending and unbending of the limbs pumps the lymphatic system, helping to eliminate stagnation and boost and strengthen the immune system.

The rhythmic movements of the limbs towards and away from the body cause blood flow to increase to and from the heart, strengthening the major arteries and veins. Most heart conditions relate to hardening and blockage in these vessels, and not to the heart muscle itself (unless it is already damaged). Thus t'ai chi can play a major role in helping to avoid heart conditions. The Taoists consider that simply causing the heart to beat faster does not yield any great long-term benefits (and may even cause overuse and eventually exhaustion of the heart muscle) but that freeing up and strengthening the arteries and veins of the heart is most important. The use of internal spiralling actions throughout the body also assists in blood circulation, as it

Right A yoga posture showing the use of maximum stretching and the locking open of the joints of the arms and legs. Many yoga postures are difficult for most people to achieve.

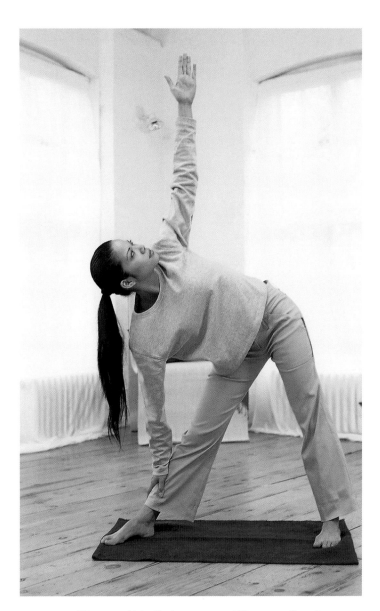

causes a gentle, rhythmic squeezing and release of all the tissues. This can enormously benefit those with impaired circulation, a common condition in the elderly and those with sedentary lifestyles. Increased blood flow naturally benefits the brain, fostering mental acuity and alertness.

The Taoists say that "the chi is the commander of the blood" and this is one reason why energetic work surpasses purely physical work: when chi flows smoothly the blood does too, fully nourishing the entire body. The rhythmic compression and release of the internal organs, combined with internal twistings that can reduce adhesions of the organs to the ribs and spine, cause proper blood and fluid flow to be restored, and can greatly enhance organ function. The release of tension within the nervous system allows the muscles to relax; combined with the use of specific physical alignments, this can allow the correction of spinal and joint misalignments, healing many back, neck and joint problems. The gentle stretching and release of ligaments and tendons greatly assist in this. For the elderly and those with bad balance, t'ai chi develops a much greater physical stability, helping to avoid falls. It can give all practitioners a sense of having their feet firmly on the ground, and this has a correspondingly stabilizing mental and emotional effect.

All these actions, combined with the direct mental manipulation of chi, cause the energy of the body to become free and strong. In terms of physical health, this particularly benefits the internal organs and the glandular system. Medical studies have proved that regular t'ai chi practice boosts immune system function and endocrine levels relating to every system of the body. T'ai chi has also been shown to be effective in lowering high blood pressure, mainly due to its effect on the deep veins and arteries.

The effect of t'ai chi practice on the nervous system is harder to measure, but it is renowned for making practitioners feel "alive" and physically relaxed. It can also help to restore lost or diminished nerve function, for example following surgery or accidental damage.

T'AI CHI AND YOGA
Yoga, a physical and energetic self-development practice originating in ancient India, is also a type of internal art, and is very effective if properly taught and applied. Where t'ai chi and yoga differ is in their approaches and methods: whereas t'ai chi seeks to find stillness in movement, enabling the continuous flow and transformation of energy within the practitioner, yoga uses fixed postures to "dam up" and release energy in certain energetic centres. Whereas t'ai chi focuses on releasing the nervous system and the inside of the body, yoga focuses on stretching and releasing its outer

structure. The result is that yoga practitioners often have greater physical flexibility than t'ai chi practitioners, but the latter often have more relaxed bodies and nervous systems. They also have superior balance and movement abilities, and of course martial abilities, which are absent from yoga.

Yoga is an excellent practice for those with healthy spines and joints, but it should be approached with caution if problems exist in these areas, as it has a more "fiery" approach than t'ai chi and may not always fully take into account existing structural problems. The t'ai chi approach – of relaxing and releasing the body and always working within current limitations – is arguably superior if you wish to heal back, neck and joint problems.

SELF-HEALING
To list the many and various health benefits that regular t'ai chi practice can bring would take up many pages; to some extent every medical condition can be improved by it. This is because when the energy, blood, fluid and organ functions of the body are improved, it can begin the process of healing itself. T'ai chi is not a miracle cure, but in many areas t'ai chi practice can indeed work wonders. It is really a life-long health insurance policy.

The Mind–Body Connection

The Taoists consider that body and mind are not only related but inseparable. Of the eight energetic bodies that make up a human being, the physical body is the most gross, and the emotional, mental and psychic bodies are progressively more subtle and expansive, but all are interpenetrating and interrelated. Therefore anything that occurs within one level will have an impact on other levels as well.

In general, the more subtle bodies have a greater and more immediate effect on the less subtle, and vice versa: while your mental state has a great and immediate effect on your physical state, your physical state will not necessarily affect your mental state quite so immediately. The Taoists were not alone in observing this mind–body interrelationship; many traditions, both Eastern and Western, use different terms to describe it. The key principle is that mind and body are inseparable.

So-called "Western" thinking about mind and body is actually relatively modern, and can be seen as stemming from the work of the philosopher René Descartes in the 17th century. The key phrase in Cartesian dualism is: "I think, therefore I am." In other words, the thinking mind is set apart from all other aspects of being, including the physical body. The implications of this philosophy extend to our attitudes to the world around us – we see the world as separate from ourselves and no longer believe ourselves to be an integral part of nature. A pre-Cartesian attitude could

be expressed as "I feel, therefore I am," encompassing our whole experience of existence, not just the mental aspect. Prior to Descartes, Western philosophy was not so very different to Eastern traditions in this respect.

SCIENCE AND CHI

Many people now live in industrialized societies, the very foundations of which are based on Cartesian thinking. This permeates all aspects of our lives, especially science and medicine. Scientists and "Western" doctors are taught that all phenomena that exist can be measured and quantified, and if something cannot be measured it does not exist. This is highly relevant to the study of t'ai chi and the internal arts, because they are based on the existence of chi energy. Chi cannot be directly measured with scientific instruments, and will probably never be scientifically "validated". The reason for this is that chi relates to consciousness itself – it is a living force that can be felt and manipulated by the mind, but has no objective existence. This makes it no less real than a radio wave, but it exists in relation to our living bodies and our minds, rather than in the external world.

If we accept that Cartesian dualism is false, the fact that we can feel chi but not measure it does not invalidate its existence, any more than we would claim that our thoughts or emotions do not exist. Ultimately, from both a Taoist and Buddhist perspective, everything manifests from emptiness, and therefore nothing possesses concrete existence anyway. The branch of Western science called quantum physics entirely agrees with this, and goes so far as to state that phenomena exist only in relation to conscious observation.

BODY AND MIND IN T'AI CHI

The Taoists developed methods of working with the mind and body together; t'ai chi is one of those methods. In terms of the eight energy bodies, all energy could be considered to be some form of chi, but for the purposes of understanding

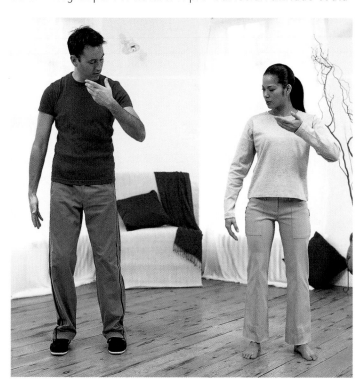

Left The practice of t'ai chi and chi gung is about learning to feel rather than think. With time, you will gain direct and definite experience of your chi energy.

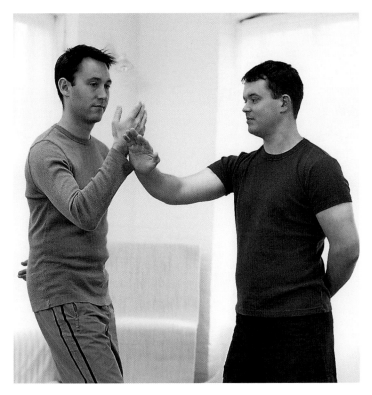

Above Learning to relax and develop open awareness while doing push hands practice with a partner.

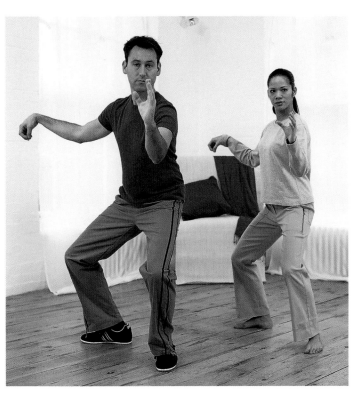

Above Moving into a meditation point within the Wu style Form – integrating meditation with movement.

t'ai chi the word "chi" is used here to refer specifically to the second of the energy bodies – the energy that circulates through the physical body and immediately surrounds it (the "aura"). The word "mind" means the intent or "i" (pronounced "yee"). This is the basic intent of your consciousness, which is involved in any action you perform. Often the simpler the action, the clearer intent is: picking up a teacup involves the intention to do that, but does not normally involve any logical thought process – you simply do it, rather than thinking about how or why you are doing it – whereas more complex actions may start to involve your thinking mind. Using the mind to move chi refers to pure intent and not to an analytical process of thinking about moving chi. It is intent – "i" – that connects with chi; the thinking mind actually hinders the process. This is a crucial point for t'ai chi practitioners to understand and develop. An oft-quoted phrase, "No 'i', no chi," means that if the intent is not present and clear the chi energy will not move as desired. Developing this clear intent, free of discursive thought processes, is a gradual process, but one that yields extraordinary results, both in chi development and in the development of a highly relaxed, yet simultaneously highly focused, mind.

T'ai chi works with the body, chi and mind at the same time, each component augmenting the development of the others in a synergistic way. The alignments and actions of the body assist the flow of chi. The flow of chi helps the body to relax and energize, and the mind to become still. A still and focused mind can move chi at will, allowing the body to remain relaxed. T'ai chi practice should always involve body, chi and mind – take one component out and the circle is

broken. While you may wish to emphasize or concentrate on one or two aspects in your training, you should always remember that this is just preparation for the performance of t'ai chi with your body, chi and mind working in harmony.

Your current experience will most likely not be that of the total integration of your body, chi and mind. If you perceive these aspects of your being to be separate, you will find it easier to refer to them that way for the purposes of working with them – and then as you become more experienced, seek to connect them and start to reintegrate them. Eventually, you may reach a stage of t'ai chi practice where they feel as if they are one – this is the point at which t'ai chi can become a truly mystical experience. This experience is not reserved for Taoist sages: it is potentially available to every ordinary man and woman.

THE MIND AND EMOTIONS

T'ai chi is superb as a relaxation practice. The emphasis on dropping and settling chi causes the mind to relax, and leads to increasing mental stillness. This in turn allows the nervous system to relax and release, which generates physical relaxation. The slow, rhythmic movements provide an antidote to frenetic daily activity and act as a metronome for your internal rhythms, allowing you to slow down and relax mentally. In addition, the physical movements and internal work allow for the release of bound emotional tensions, bringing about a sense of inner peace and emotional "smoothness". T'ai chi can develop a relaxed mental focus while fully exercising both sides of the brain with the coordination of simultaneous movement on the left and right sides of the body.

The Use of Meditation in T'ai Chi

T'ai chi is often described as a form of "moving meditation". Its mind–body synergy makes it a practice that is inherently meditative in nature. However, if we look more deeply at Taoist self-development practice we will see that t'ai chi is not in itself a meditation practice, but that it can be used in conjunction with meditation techniques. These techniques can then be incorporated into t'ai chi to make it a true moving meditation.

The common view of meditation is that it mainly consists of a practice that leads to relaxation, especially of the mind. It is usually assumed to be something that involves sitting motionless with the eyes closed. Both statements are true, but they do not give a complete picture of what meditation is. In the Taoist tradition, you are really practising meditation only when you are working with the energies of your consciousness, to transform blockage and tension in your emotional, mental, psychic and higher bodies. Simply becoming calmer is not meditation. However, this stillness is a prerequisite for being able to travel deeper within yourself and resolve tensions at these more subtle levels. T'ai chi practice can develop a degree of inner stillness as the foundation for deeper meditation practices. Some of these practices can be applied while doing t'ai chi: this then becomes t'ai chi meditation.

The Taoists recognize five modes of practice, relating to the basic activities of life: sitting, moving, standing, lying down and having sex. None of these modes is inherently superior to the others, but certain practices are easier to apply in certain modes. Sitting, for instance, facilitates

inwardly focused meditation practice; while standing facilitates practice relating to your physical and chi body. Once a practice has been well applied in the easiest mode for it, it is applied in all other modes. Inwardly focused practice is best learned sitting but is later applied during all the other activities, including t'ai chi form practice. The deeper Taoist meditation practices must be learned directly from a teacher, but some simple and effective practices are detailed in this book.

NORMAL T'AI CHI PRACTICE

T'ai chi has many different aspects; every practitioner will find their own personal areas of interest, and focus on them. It is possible to develop your body and chi, and achieve a degree of stillness, without venturing into the realms of meditation – there have been many t'ai chi masters who were not particularly interested in meditation or spiritual practice. This is a personal choice. True meditation practice can be a bumpy ride: to resolve deep-seated emotional, mental and psychic tensions you have to confront them nakedly. The phrase "face your demons" is apt. Not

Far left Meditation practice sitting in the lotus position. This is a useful and very stable position, but difficult for many people.

Left Sitting on a chair can be equally effective for meditation, and is more comfortable and familiar to most Westerners.

Below Meditating lying down allows for greater relaxation of the body, although there is a tendency to become drowsy in this position.

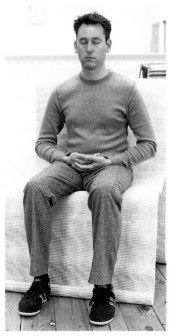

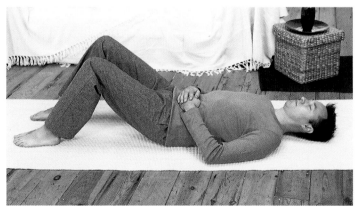

Right The Wu style posture "single whip". This posture and the posture "fan through the back" help to open the central energetic channel. These meditation points in the form enable the practitioner to release any tensions in his or her mind and energy into empty space, before continuing with the form.

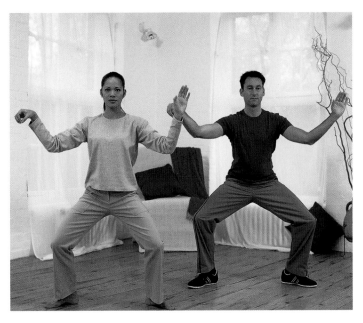

everybody wants to do this, or feels ready to undertake this kind of work. For many, to become a little more relaxed and a lot healthier is enough.

Even without engaging in deeper meditation practices, the mind and chi work inherent in normal t'ai chi practice can have a profound effect on your mental and emotional world. It has a powerful effect in three specific areas: the nervous system (including the brain); the glands (endocrine system); and the main internal organs. Your nervous system is freed of tension and strengthened by practice. This reduces internal "noise" (a key symptom of prolonged and unresolved stress), bringing about a quietening of the mind and a sense of mental peace. Your glands are allowed to function smoothly, as they are boosted where deficient and calmed where overactive. The effects of this are very great, as the hormones secreted by the glands have an enormously powerful effect on the mind and emotions. For instance, overactive and "edgy" adrenal glands will mean that you are always "revved-up" mentally and emotionally. The main organs of the body relate to the basic "lower" emotions such as anger and grief, and imbalances here will cause corresponding emotional imbalances that will affect the corresponding organ. T'ai chi practice can break the cycle and restore balance.

THE DEEPER PRACTICES

One of the ways in which t'ai chi works to achieve internal transformations is through repetitive and rhythmic external motions. This is known in many traditions: Zen Buddhist monks, for example, are often given the task of polishing rice or washing dishes all day for many months. As they do this, their minds turn inwards and start to process their internal tensions, eventually releasing them and achieving stillness. The rhythmic motions of t'ai chi can have the same effect when linked to meditation practice.

In the context of the repetitive external activity in t'ai chi, meditation techniques can be applied, "dissolving" tensions inwardly, back into the emptiness that underlies all existence. This inner dissolving is distinct from the practice of outer dissolving, where the practitioner releases blockages in chi (relating to places in the physical body) outwardly until they become neutralized. Inner dissolving practice is applied to all the systems of the physical body, including the organs, glands, spinal cord and brain. Emotional, mental and psychic tensions can be stored in the physical body, and these can be accessed and released with

Right Push hands practice can provide a "reality check" for your levels of emotional smoothness and stillness.

the aid of the various postures and movements of t'ai chi. Eventually the inner dissolving practices allow for the practitioner to enter the central point (called t'ai chi) where there is no distinction between yin and yang, everything is inherently empty, and their true nature is revealed. A phrase used to denote this in relation to t'ai chi chuan practice is "stillness in movement, movement in stillness": stillness (yin) and movement (yang) become inseparable and indistinguishable from one another. This phrase has significant implications for meditation and spiritual practice.

PUSH HANDS AND MEDITATION

T'ai chi push hands practice is a very useful method for moving towards this state, as the two-person work provides a yardstick against which to measure and develop your ability to be truly relaxed and truly present while engaged in external movement and internal energetic work. If you become angry, fearful or upset when pushed by your partner, you may not be as emotionally relaxed as you think.

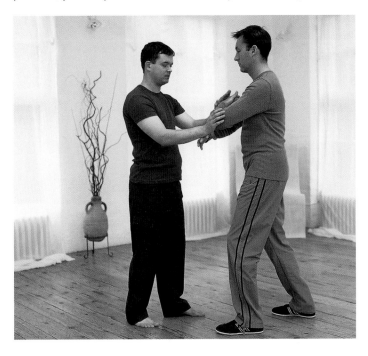

Healing Back and Neck Problems

Many people take up t'ai chi because they are suffering from stress and are looking for a relaxation practice, or are seeking long-term relief from back, neck and joint pain. These two problems often go hand-in-hand: stress generally leads to physical stiffness and pain, and prolonged spinal and joint pain almost always causes stress. As we age, our bodies contract. T'ai chi can help alleviate this tendency and enable mobility well into old age.

Occupations such as desk-bound office work may cause both stress and musculoskeletal problems. They are by far the most common health complaints in the developed world, and entire industries have grown up around them. From pharmaceuticals to relaxation tapes, from magnetic mattresses to on-site massage, there are hundreds of different "solutions" on offer. While some are more effective than others, most tend to focus on either back pain or stress, but not fully on both. T'ai chi is truly unsurpassed in helping to solve both of these problems simultaneously.

Spinal and joint problems can be roughly divided into two types: tension and misalignment. Like everything else relating to t'ai chi, neither really exists in isolation. Tension can be defined as tightness in the muscles, fascia and "sinews" (ligaments and tendons). A simple tension might be a knot (twisted muscle fibres) in the back muscles, which can be relieved, at least temporarily, by massage. Misalignment can be defined as imbalances in the skeletal structure, and misplacement of the ligaments and tendons.

A misalignment might take the form of one or more spinal vertebrae that are subluxated (twisted out of their proper place), or a tendon that does not run smoothly through the proper groove over a joint. Misalignments are typically treated by manipulation, such as that performed by chiropractors and osteopaths. These "adjustments" physically move the vertebrae back into their proper alignments. However, the vertebrae rarely stay there, but often return to misalignment. The reason for this also explains why t'ai chi is so effective at providing lasting correction of spinal and joint misalignments.

THE SOLUTION

Some approaches to back, neck and joint problems focus mainly on strengthening the relevant muscles. Strengthening healthy, unknotted muscles around well-aligned skeletal structures is fine, and can help to support the body. However, strengthening tense and knotted muscles surrounding misaligned vertebrae and joints is not

Below The spinal alignments of t'ai chi encourage good posture, helping to reduce the likelihood of future back and neck problems.

Below A key part of t'ai chi alignments is learning to regain space in the neck vertebrae and open the occiput at the base of the skull.

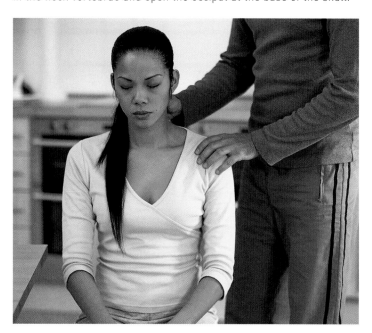

Right As an arm rises in t'ai chi, the shoulder blade drops down the back like a counterweight, avoiding tension in the shoulders and helping to release shoulder, neck and upper back problems.

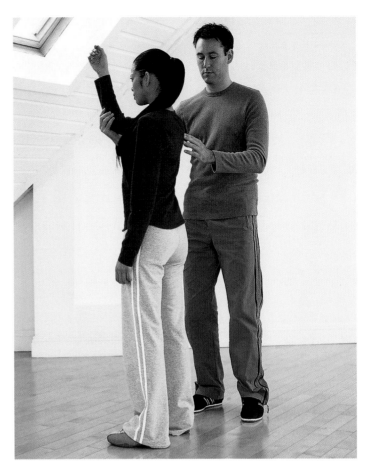

fine: it will simply strengthen the problem itself, locking it more firmly into the body. Instead, you need release. You need to release the tensions that are causing muscles to be tight and pulling skeletal structures out of alignment.

Most people with spinal and joint misalignments do not have abnormal bone structure: the building blocks are not misshapen, just badly stacked. The skeleton cannot hold itself up alone. It is held up, and aligned, by the muscles attached to the bones. When they do not pull evenly or correctly on the skeleton, they will pull parts of it out of alignment. As a result, nerves will become pinched and there will be pain. Muscles do not have minds of their own; they act only in relation to the nerve signals they are given. If a muscle is "misbehaving" and pulling the spine out of alignment, it is because there is an incorrect nerve signal to that muscle. The nerves pattern the muscles – and chi patterns the nerves. When the flow of chi is not smooth and correctly patterned, the nerve signal will also not be smooth and correctly patterned, and the muscles will contract abnormally. This is why adjustment of the bones tends not to result in permanent relief: the muscles simply pull the bones out of alignment again. In order to restore the whole system to balance, the chi patterns of the body need to be made smooth again. Normal muscle function will result, and the muscles will hold the skeleton in its natural and correct alignment. This principle also applies to pain resulting from muscular tension, which restricts blood flow and pinches local nerves.

THE METHOD

T'ai chi practice heals these problems by relaxing the nervous system, smoothing and balancing the flow of chi, and gently stretching and releasing the internal and external muscles. The specific skeletal alignments of t'ai chi then allow the bones and joints to fall into their proper locations.

Tense muscles tend to lack sufficient blood flow, and this is a major cause of pain. The inward and outward movements of t'ai chi gently stretch and compress the muscles, "wringing" blood through them. The ligaments and tendons are gently stretched and released, and this restores lost flexibility and length, as well as healthy chi flow through the tissues. Tight, shortened ligaments and tendons are often a cause of problems around the joints. The spiralling actions of t'ai chi are a key factor in their release.

The fascia – a thin sheet of tissue that wraps around your entire body – is released through proper t'ai chi movement. When tight, it can act like a strait jacket, constricting the deeper muscles and joints. T'ai chi effectively removes this strait jacket, allowing access to the deeper levels of the body. Once joint pulsing has been learned, the opening and closing of all the joints from the inside dramatically increases the amount of synovial fluid, chi and space in the joints. T'ai chi is known for combating arthritis. Where there are spinal misalignments, pulsing gives vertebrae the space they need to return to proper alignment. In the case of a slipped disc, this will remove the pressure on the disc so that it is no longer forced out of the intervertebral space.

Where lower back (lumbar) problems exist, t'ai chi's emphasis on releasing and working with the kwa (the groin area at the front of the pelvis) will allow the pelvis as a whole to release and realign, releasing and stabilizing the sacrum, misalignment of which is often the source of lower back problems. Wu style t'ai chi places a strong emphasis on the kwa, and is known for healing lower back complaints in particular. In the case of upper back and neck problems, the release of the shoulder blades, called the "hidden joints of the body" by the Taoists, allows for the release of the entire area. Another common cause of musculoskeletal problems is the weakening of the insertion points where the muscles attach to the bones. These can tear away, resulting – in extreme cases – in complete loss of use of the muscle. Surgery is then the only recourse. T'ai chi stretches and strengthens these insertion points so that the problem is less likely to occur.

T'ai chi has much to offer in terms of health, longevity and well-being, but the most compelling reason for many people to start learning it is its superb record in healing back, neck and joint problems. Many Western doctors now recommend it to their patients for exactly this reason.

Energizing

At times, many people lack the energy they need to cope with the demands of everyday life. This feeling of low energy can result in a lack of enthusiasm for life, a feeling that it is all "too much". At the extreme, it can lead to despondency and even depression. This is a very common problem, especially for people who lead stressful lives. Often that stress causes insomnia, which prevents sufferers from replenishing their energy during the night.

Chronic tiredness is very common in people who have sedentary occupations, such as office workers. They are not expending large amounts of physical energy every day, yet are far more tired and de-energized than those who do expend energy in physical work. In terms of an "energy in/energy out" equation this seems to make no sense: if you are using less energy surely you should have more available. However, there is a factor at work that is the single biggest cause of most fatigue syndromes: blockage.

BLOCKAGE
The energetic system and its channels are like a network of water pipes connected to a reservoir. If the pipes are open and clear, water can flow through and out of them as fast as fresh water flows into them from the reservoir. You are constantly refilling your reservoir of energy from the air you breathe, the food you eat, and also from external sources such as sunlight and moonlight. If the pipes are partly blocked, however, then no matter how much water is in the reservoir, you will only get a trickle out of the pipes. Clear

the blockage, and the normal flow is restored, to be put to whatever use you choose. The desk-bound office worker may feel more exhausted than the bricklayer because his or her energy has stagnated. As with slowly moving water, which allows silt to accumulate, the channels have become blocked. Blockage can also occur for other reasons, such as physical damage to the body, or mental and emotional tension, but whatever the cause, the methods used to restore normal energetic flows are more or less the same. Also, you would focus on healing the root cause of the blockage, including harmful habits.

T'ai chi practice opens the energy channels of the body, both by correcting the physical misalignments and tensions that cause blockage and by directly opening the channels and causing chi to flow through them, thus "washing away" blockage. Every posture in the t'ai chi form causes chi to move in patterns that benefit specific channels and centres in the body. The constantly flowing nature of the form itself encourages chi to move freely where it may be stagnant. The mental and emotional relaxation that practice brings

Left Releasing chi energy in a posture from the Wu style long form. The martial origins of t'ai chi are clearly visible in this movement.

Below The storing (left) and release (right) of energy in the Wu style t'ai chi posture of "ji" (push). Note the compression and release of the kwa area at the front of the pelvis.

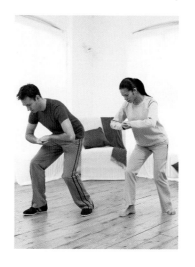

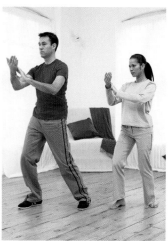

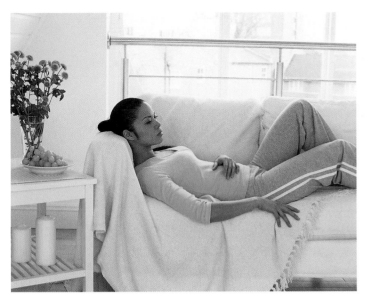

"unfreezes" chi, which can become frozen due to stress. Any physical exercise will help reduce chi stagnation, but because t'ai chi operates on a deeper level, and more directly with the energetic system as well as with the mind, it brings proportionally greater results in this area.

HOW IT WORKS

There is a specific process that has the greatest effect in removing blockage: the gathering and releasing of energy. T'ai chi is based mainly on yin/yang theory, and the ebb and flow of its movements perfectly reflect this. Performing a t'ai chi form (and push hands), you move from yin postures and movements to yang postures and movements in a continuous, alternating flow. On a physical level, simply moving the arms towards your body, then away, then towards your body again, forms a cycle from yin to yang and back to yin again. You also open and close your joints, compress and release internal spaces in the body, bow and release your spine, spiral your energy out and back, and allow your mind – your intent – to go outwards and then inwards. All these actions take the form of a yin/yang cycle, as in the t'ai chi symbol. When you near the completion of yin, you start becoming yang, and vice versa, never stopping.

The continuous pulsing action of your body, your energy and your mind mirrors the pulsation that everything in the universe, from atoms to galaxies, constantly undergoes. Pulsation is life: stop pulsing (your breathing, your heartbeat) and you will die. This is an example of the microcosmic/macrocosmic nature of t'ai chi practice: with it you seek to integrate more fully with, and reactivate, this natural pulsation within yourself. As a result you begin to feel more alive.

BUILDING YOUR RESERVES

Having removed the blockages in your energetic system, and regained the energy that should naturally be available to you, you can set about increasing your core reserves of chi. There are several reasons why you would want to do this: by increasing your reserves, you also increase the

energy immediately available to you; with a bigger reservoir you can draw more at any moment; you can sustain an output of energy for longer without becoming "drained"; and you have emergency reserves for those times, such as illness or great stress, when you really need extra energy. In terms of jing, this means that your post-birth jing is strong enough that you need not tap into your pre-birth jing, even in extreme circumstances.

During t'ai chi practice, you would choose to release proportionally more chi than you gather in order to eliminate stagnation in your chi. Once this has been achieved, you would seek to gather proportionally more than you release in order to build your reserves. The balance between gathering and releasing may vary from day to day, or from month to month, as the activities you take part in, and the condition of your energy and mind, will vary. Being sensitive to your internal state is an important skill to develop. As a general rule, you should seek to gather and release energy in a ratio of about 80:20, in order to build your reserves.

Chi that is gathered is stored in the lower tantien. This then naturally replenishes jing, which is stored in the kidneys. There are many elderly t'ai chi practitioners who, in their seventies and even beyond, possess the energy, mental acuity, sexual function and physical mobility of people half their age. These elderly practitioners also enjoy the mental, emotional and spiritual peace that should naturally develop with age, but so often does not. This is a direct result of the t'ai chi principle of regaining the natural freedom of body, energy and mind that we possess as babies. Observe a baby moving and you will see all of the t'ai chi principles at work.

Below A relaxed and healthy flow of chi energy enables you to enjoy life more fully, and it opens up your innate creative abilities that have the potential to make life truly fulfilling.

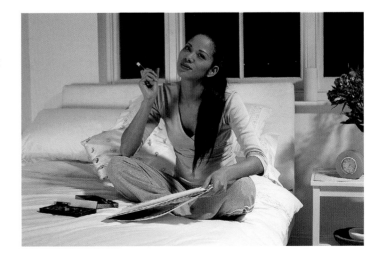

Reducing Stress and Stilling the Mind

Stress has become an almost universal complaint in modern society, to the extent that many Western doctors consider stress-related illness the "number one killer". In terms of costs resulting from lost working days and loss of skilled employees due to "burn-out", stress is a major problem for all developed nations. Stress negatively affects all the body's systems, and has been proven to dramatically reduce immune system function.

The costs to the individual suffering from chronic stress – loss of employment, relationships, and physical and psychological health – are compelling reasons to take action to reduce this burden.

It is natural to experience stress, whether physical or psychological, simply as a consequence of living. Problems arise only when stress is not released following the event that caused it, but retained within the body and mind; when new stressful events take place, tension begins to accumulate. Stress usually becomes chronic for one of two reasons: either the person is not able to relax following a stressful event, or so many stressful events occur in succession that there is simply no time to "unwind", and each event increases the stress burden. Either way, the solution is to learn to relax, and to be able to do so quickly and easily.

HEAVEN AND EARTH

T'ai chi practice works on the symptoms of stress, such as "frozen" chi and tensions within the body and nervous system. The feedback effect this causes allows for greater relaxation and, in turn, further release of tension. It also involves energetic work that directly causes the mind to relax and become still, immediately dissolving stress. The principles behind this work are very simple.

Two primordial flows of energy pass through the body in opposite directions: from heaven to earth, and from earth to heaven. They flow from above the body downwards and out through the feet, and vice versa, through the feet, up the body and out through the crown of the head. It is said by the Taoists that the energy of heaven descends and causes the energy of earth to respond (and rise), bringing about physical existence. The downward flow, yin in nature, allows for the release of tension and blockage throughout the system. The nature of the downward flow is like water, which seeks the lowest point and flows down without effort. The upward, yang, flow allows you to become energized and to maintain a physical body. It also has a "spiritualizing" aspect. Its nature is like fire, which leaps upwards and constantly seeks to move. In terms of reducing stress and

stilling the mind, it is the downward flow that is of paramount importance.

The Taoists have a saying, "The brain eats the body", which refers to the propensity of an overactive brain (the thinking mind) to monopolize the energy available. When this happens there is insufficient energy available for the rest of the body, and it suffers as a consequence. The brain is being "greedy" and damaging the body. Occupations that

Below Using Taoist breathing meditation to release tension and start approaching stillness of mind. This is a powerful method of dealing with accumulated stress.

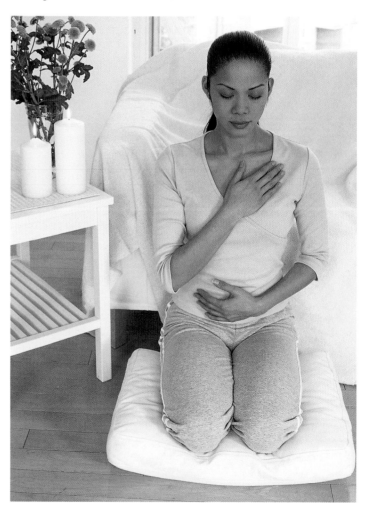

principally involve mental work can result in the overactivity of the brain. Once it has drawn a lot of energy upwards into itself, that energy tends to become stuck there. The result can be likened to a car engine with a stuck throttle: it revs out of control. This is a major cause of insomnia and anxiety. If you can get the excess energy to drop back into the body, the brain will calm down again.

Of the two major flows of energy, the upward flow is very easy to activate. The downward flow tends not to occur so readily in most people. It is relatively easy to become agitated and stay that way, with accompanying feelings of energy rising to your head, but much harder to become calm and stay calm. The common phrases "being grounded" and "being down to earth" perfectly express the importance of the downward flow of energy in achieving a relaxed and calm mind. It is important to understand that it is not the rising of energy itself that causes anxiety, but that energy becoming stuck in the upper body and brain, because there is not an equal, balancing downward flow of chi. The downward flow not only opens but also strengthens the channels, ready to handle the power of the fire-like, yang upward flow. For this reason, it is best to be cautious about undertaking any practices that heavily emphasize the upward flow before you have stabilized the downward flow. If this is not done, energetic "burn-out" can result, sometimes with serious consequences for mind and body.

T'ai chi practice heavily emphasizes developing the downward flow (in the initial stages), and regaining the ability to activate it fully at will. Ideally, this flow should be constant and automatic, and with practice it can become so. The practice of ba gua zhang, which tends to create a strong upward spiralling of energy, is best undertaken after some training in t'ai chi, or at least standing practice, so that the downward flow is continuously activated. (This is one of the factors that makes ba gua more difficult to learn than t'ai chi.) T'ai chi practitioners talk of growing a "root". Just like the roots of a tree, this means getting your chi to sink and connect into the ground beneath your feet. When this happens, not only do you clear blockages in your energy channels, and still your mind, you also connect fully with the flow of energy upwards from the ground, which can then move freely and smoothly through your open channels. This is a major source of power in the internal martial arts, so activating the downward energy flow is the key to utilizing the upward flow fully as well. The core practice for activating and developing the downward flow is standing practice, called zhan zhuang, or "standing like a tree". It is important to start with standing postures that emphasize the downward energy flow.

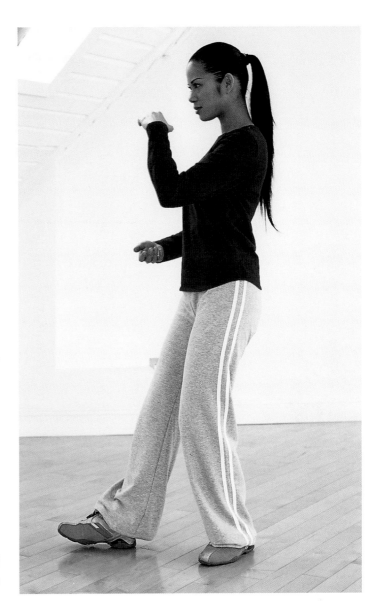

Above The "yin releasing" posture from the Wu form can be used as a standing posture to help release tension. It emphasizes the dropping of chi down the yin channels of the front of the body.

DROPPING THE MIND

As well as activating the downward, yin energy flow, in t'ai chi and chi gung practice you develop the ability to drop your mind into your lower tantien. This means that your awareness moves fully into that part of your body, where that energy centre is located. Found approximately four fingers' breadth below the navel, and on the central channel deep within the body, the lower tantien is the main energetic centre of the physical body. When your awareness moves into this centre, two things happen: your mind becomes still, and it connects with the chi of your entire body, awakening it. All movement in t'ai chi originates in the lower tantien, and your mind should be present there throughout your practice. As a result, you will have progressively deeper experiences of stillness, during which tensions and stress will dissolve and release effortlessly. The experience of "monkey mind", where the mind jumps constantly from one thought to another, will subside, and you will develop truly relaxed focus, your mind still and yet fully aware.

Balancing the Emotions

There are times when we feel that we have become ruled by our emotions, losing perspective and clarity with regard to the situation in which we find ourselves. The emotions that can overtake us vary widely, but the effect is the same: we can find ourselves acting in ways that are not beneficial to ourselves or others. A classic example would be becoming overcome by anger and saying or doing something that we later come to regret.

Strong emotions can blind us to what is actually happening, causing us to overreact or act inappropriately. From a Taoist perspective, emotions themselves are not enemies or things to be eliminated; it is a question of balance. We are not robots, we are human beings, and human beings have emotions. Those beginning meditation often ask, "If I eliminate my emotions, what will remain of my personality?" This question reflects a common misunderstanding of the process of working with emotions in the context of meditation and t'ai chi practice. We are seeking not to become unfeeling, but to achieve a state where we are not slaves to our emotions – where we can fully experience them without becoming conditioned by them. As a result we can discover our true personality, rather than one based on our individual emotional imbalances. This true personality is not only far stronger than the "imbalance personality" but is likely to be far more attractive to other people, especially those who are similarly balanced emotionally.

A person who seems angry and aggressive may actually have a true personality of great kindness and compassion, concealed (even from themselves) by the obvious imbalances.

If our emotional energy is truly balanced we will always experience emotions that are appropriate to a situation. When the situation that brought about that emotional experience ends, the emotional experience will also end. Without this balance we might, for example, get angry about something inconsequential, feeling overcome by rage, and then continue to feel angry after the situation has ended. This principle applies to any of the emotions: excessive sadness, for instance, can develop into depression.

THE EMOTIONS AND THE ORGANS

Chinese medical theory is very much concerned with the emotions, and it is considered that the energies of each of the main organs generate the emotions. This is related to Five Element theory, in which each element, or phase of energy, has its expression in a particular emotion. Each organ also houses an aspect of the shen, or spirit. In simple form, the correspondences are:

Heart
Fire; joy (enjoyment of life); pure consciousness
Spleen
Earth; caring (for yourself and others); intention ("i")
Lungs
Metal; grief (letting go); "earthly" spirit
Kidneys
Water; fear (self-reflection and re-evaluation); willpower
Liver
Wood; anger (ability to take necessary action); "heavenly" spirit

Each of the emotions has its proper time and place for expression, and its proper function. None is considered negative in itself: even anger is beneficial if it is applied correctly, for the correct reason – for instance, by a mother protecting her child. Joy provides the spark of life; grief is

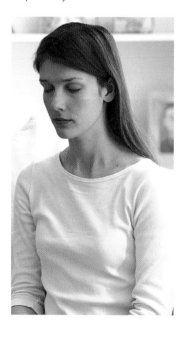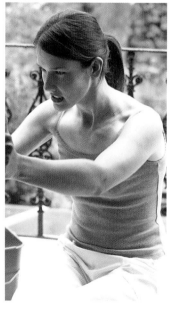

Above Balancing the emotions is about avoiding the two extremes of emotionlessness and of excessive emotionality. A balance between these two allows for the normal expression of emotion, without the damaging effects of suppression or overindulgence.

Right Practising Cloud Hands chi gung. The t'ai chi principles embodied in this exercise represent the Taoist philosophy of balance in every aspect of your being: physical, energetic and mental/emotional balance.

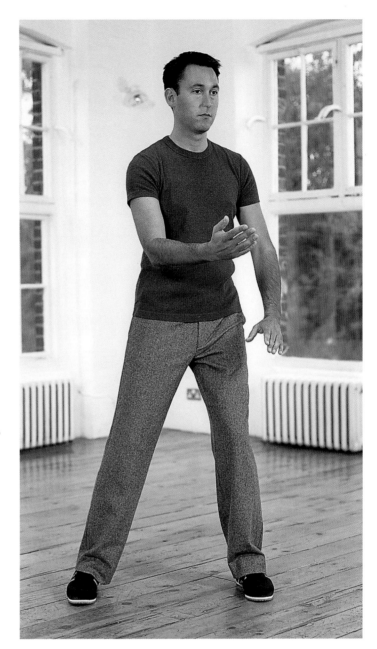

required if we are to let go of people or things we have lost; caring for ourselves and others is essential; and it is through sadness that we know withdrawal and change is necessary. What is important is that these emotions are not inappropriately expressed or prolonged. Excess and deficiency of the emotions are equally harmful: excessive grief is an inability to let go, and becomes attachment, which often leads to anger; excessive caring becomes obsession, neediness and smothering; excessive joy becomes mania. Deficient joy becomes lifelessness, while deficient or unexpressed anger becomes frustration, and then depression. These are just a few examples: it is very useful to contemplate the beneficial and harmful aspects of all the emotions for yourself, and how they apply to you.

CORRECTING IMBALANCE

When all the emotions are balanced and properly expressed, the result is a "balanced person". As a personal practice, examine your own emotional responses throughout the day, trying to be aware of where and when your emotions are balanced, and when they are out of balance. This will give you a sense of where your focus should lie in your own emotional self-development practice. Also observe your partner and friends: the emotional patterns of people with whom you choose to associate will often mirror your own (like attracts like). Often, the very realization that you are over- or under-expressing a particular emotion can lead to a shift in your mentality, and a rebalancing of that emotion. This is particularly effective where the cause of the imbalance is mainly habitual – psychological conditioning rather than an organ imbalance.

Where there is an imbalance within the organs of your body, that needs to be addressed directly, through treatment such as acupuncture and practices such as chi gung and t'ai chi. If there has been a long-term pattern of a particular emotion being excessive or deficient, there will usually be an imbalance in the corresponding organ. The organ imbalance will cause a corresponding imbalance in the manifestation of the emotion, and the excessive or deficient expression of that emotion will in turn affect the organ negatively. So whether the root cause of the imbalance is at the level of the organs or the mind, both need to be addressed, as they are mutually dependent. Most people are born with an imbalance in one of their organs – and therefore in the corresponding element – and life-long emotional patterns may be directly caused by this. You may not be able to eliminate your hereditary imbalance completely, but you can practically eliminate its impact on your life using methods such as t'ai chi practice. When you

discover what your hereditary imbalance is, it can be a life-changing revelation, in terms of not only your health but also your emotional life.

T'ai chi works to calm your nervous system and mind, and to release emotional energies ("memories") that are stuck within your body. This smooths out your overall emotional state, allowing you to work more directly with the organs to release blockage, re-energize and balance them. The calming effects of t'ai chi on the glands help to unwind the addiction to very powerful hormonal secretions that usually accompanies an emotional pattern. For instance, a person who is frequently enraged will receive a large dose of adrenalin with each "freak-out", and this adrenalin "hit" can become addictive. All the emotions trigger glandular secretions, and some are opiates stronger than heroin. In the case of strong emotions, it is necessary to relax this glandular response. T'ai chi achieves this, largely as a result of its balancing effects on all the body's chi. Meditation practice can also be applied to specific glands and organs, to further the effects.

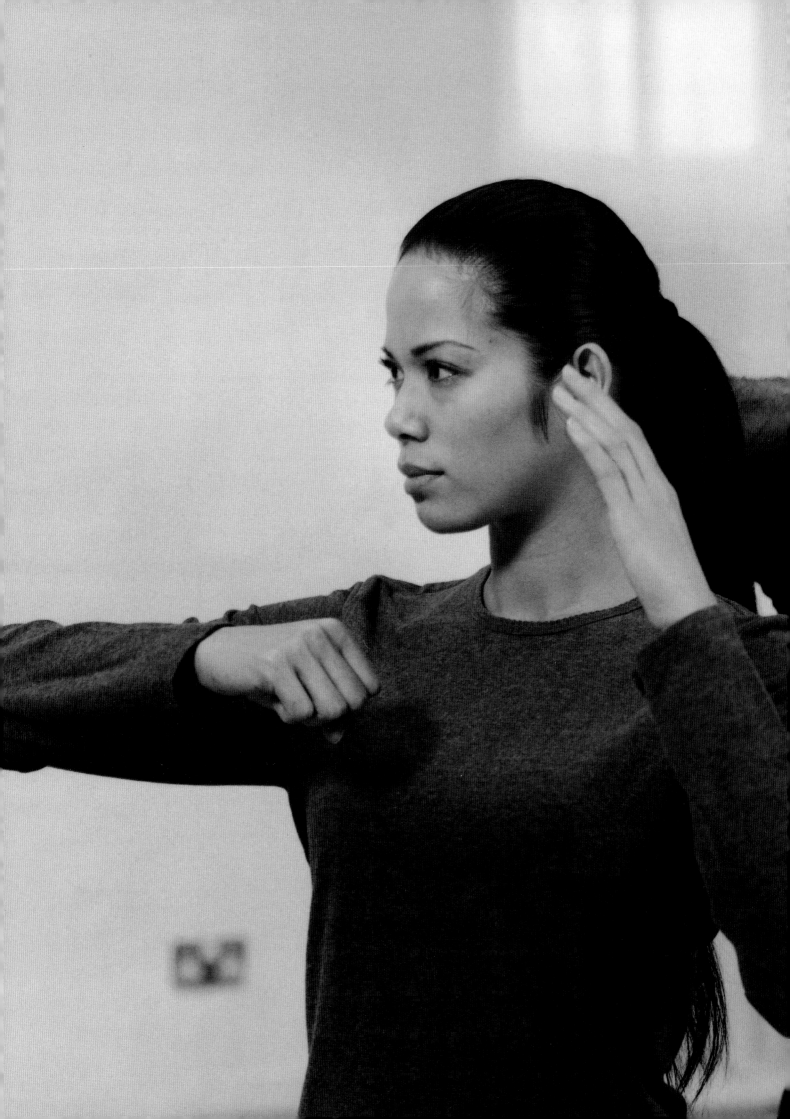

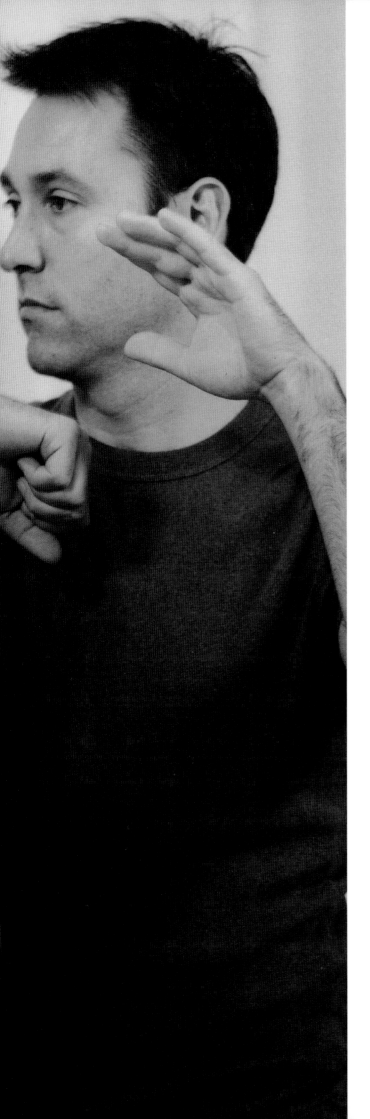

Preparation

The practical section of this book starts with the fundamental principles of t'ai chi, with an overview of the energetic system of the body and how it functions, especially in relation to t'ai chi practice. It shows the precise body alignments that allow for optimum chi flow and release of physical blockages, and how to move in accordance with t'ai chi principles, unifying all parts of the body. The section on relaxing and releasing shows how to work solo and with a partner to loosen your body and release tension. Finally, the section on Cloud Hands chi gung gives a complete chi gung practice that embodies key Taoist nei gung principles, fundamental to t'ai chi. Practised alongside the t'ai chi form, Cloud Hands will greatly enhance your understanding of t'ai chi and speed up your development as a practitioner. Cloud Hands offers many of the physical, energetic and mental/emotional benefits of t'ai chi in a simple and easy-to-learn practice.

T'ai Chi Principles

Taoist nei gung principles form the core of t'ai chi. However, because learning t'ai chi also involves learning many complex movements, it is much easier to learn nei gung principles outside t'ai chi practice itself, and then incorporate them into your t'ai chi form once you have mastered them. This is the main reason to practise secondary exercises such as those shown in this chapter.

The overriding principle in t'ai chi is to relax. This does not mean becoming floppy and collapsed, either physically or mentally, but becoming soong: a state of being unbound by any tension. A general guide is that you should use only enough muscle power to maintain the structure of your body and your postures. Feelings of strength in the body are actually indications of blockage at those places. For instance, if you raise an arm, you should use only the basic muscle power required to do that, and no more. This would be no more than about 10 per cent of your muscle power, possibly far less. When you relax this much, your chi flows very strongly through your body, and true internal power starts to manifest. However, becoming this soong is not so easy, especially for beginners. The more empty your body is, the more chi energy will flow through it. Try to keep this principle in mind at all times and it will naturally develop within you. Never get annoyed at yourself for being tense. Remember: you will not become relaxed by being tense.

ENERGETIC CHANNELS

For the practice of Wu style t'ai chi, you need to be aware of three main energetic channels in your body. The central channel runs from the crown of the head (baihui) exactly through the centre of the body on a straight line to the perineum (huiyin), and also through the bone marrow of the arms and legs. All three tantiens are located on the central channel, and this pathway is the main focus of Taoist meditation and spiritual practice.

The side channels run either side of the central channel, midway between the front and back of the body (like the central channel). As well as the central channel, Wu style t'ai chi works specifically with the side channels, and in many of the postures the hands are in alignment with them on their respective sides. The central channel is the primordial energetic pathway of the body, and is formed when the egg first divides in the womb. The side channels are formed with the next division, and from them all the other channels are spun out. Working with these deep channels affects all the other, more superficial, channels, and this is the primary reason for their emphasis.

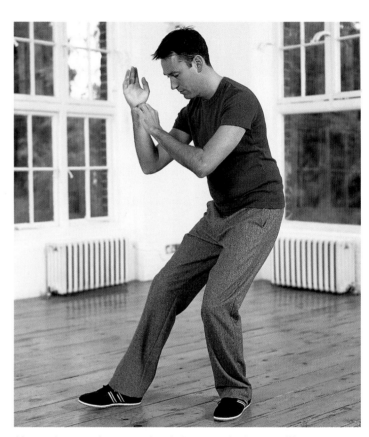

Above As you relax more deeply into your body, you will start to have a sense of moving the outside of your body from the inside, without any feeling of using external muscles to do the work.

THE TANTIENS

There are three tantiens ("elixir fields") within the body: the lower, middle and upper tantien. The lower tantien is located approximately four fingers' breadth below the navel, deep in the body on the central channel. At first, you may not be aware of your tantien, but with practice it will "wake up" and you will start to feel a sense of energy there. Initially, this may seem like a "fuzzy" area of energy, but eventually it will condense into a precise sphere, and its location will become definite.

The middle and upper tantiens are not of such primary importance in basic t'ai chi practice, as they relate more to Taoist meditation practice. The upper tantien relates more

Right Lying down, releasing the nervous system prior to beginning standing and moving practice. Note how the body is allowed to completely relax, without any holding of shape or position.

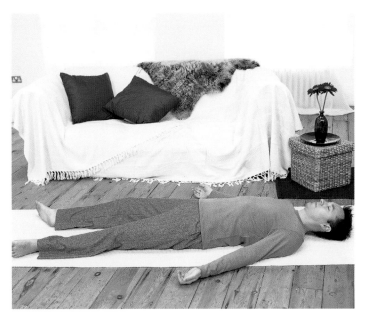

to mental and psychic energies, and the middle tantien to "pure" emotions such as compassion, and your relationship with things or ideas. It is considered the residence of true consciousness – your hsin, or "heart-mind".

All three tantiens will be benefited by normal t'ai chi practice. However, the lower tantien, being the central point for your body's chi, is of primary importance in t'ai chi.

MAJOR GATES

Specific places within the body are of major importance in allowing the free flow of chi. These are sometimes known as "energy gates", as they can close or allow chi to pass. For the purposes of t'ai chi practice, those that you should be most aware of are: the crown of the head (baihui); the occiput, where the skull sits on the neck; the base of the neck at the seventh cervical vertebra; the armpits; the centre of the midriff; the inguinal, or groin, area (kwa); the perineum (huiyin); the hollow in the ball of the foot, or Bubbling Well point (yongquan); and the centre of the palms (laogung). All the joints of the body also act as energy gates. Finally, the tailbone (coccyx), which connects spinal energy into the ground, is one of the main pathways for connecting the energies of heaven and earth within you.

THE COMFORT ZONE

As a general rule, take your practice to only about 70 per cent of your ability, whether in terms of movement or stamina. The reason for this is that you are attempting to release tensions within your body, energy and mind. If you push yourself to the limit, there will be a subconscious tension response within you. Your body will tighten automatically if it thinks it is about to be damaged by being forced open. The same applies to your mind. If you stay just outside this "danger zone", you will start relaxing on every level, and your practice will achieve its aim. If you do this, your 70 per cent will become greater in real terms.

As part of this rule of moderation, do not demand perfection of yourself. You can do only what you have the ability for, at any stage. The Taoists use the phrase "more or less" in the context of self-development practice to indicate that you should never expect to be perfect. The balance between more and less will change over time, but nobody will ever do t'ai chi perfectly.

FEELING OR VISUALIZATION

Many people assume that they should try to visualize chi flows during practice, and sometimes t'ai chi and chi gung are taught this way. However, from the perspective of the Taoist nei gung tradition, feeling is far more important than visualization. When you visualize energy flows within you they may happen accordingly, or they may not. You may simply generate sensations with your mind in a sort of self-hypnosis that misleads you. On the other hand, when you feel something happening you are in no doubt about its reality. You want to be able to forge a link between your "i" (intent) and your chi, so that you can move your chi directly without involving your thinking mind. By trying to make this connection occur, without visualizing, but being patient, you actually forge the link. Eventually you feel your chi, and are left in no doubt about what has actually occurred. This also enables you to be aware of the state of your energy, to feel blockages, and to feel your physical body more clearly. Many people have lost their natural ability to feel their own bodies and energy fully: they are over-visualized. Using this simple method, that process can be reversed.

RELEASING THE NERVOUS SYSTEM

The following technique is ideal as a preparation for practising t'ai chi or chi gung. If you are feeling stressed, the exercise may make you feel sleepy. This is normal and indicates that your nervous system is releasing tension: the more tired you feel, the more tension you have been holding within you. It is very important that you give your nervous system a chance to release before practising t'ai chi or chi gung. As you progress, you will find that your tension levels are generally lower, and this exercise is simply relaxing. Lie on your back and take a few moments to allow your mind and nervous system to settle. Then, starting at the top of your head, and moving down gradually through your body and limbs, let go of all feelings of strength and allow the floor to support you fully. Give yourself up to gravity and allow your body to become heavy, with a feeling of sinking into the ground. Take this process all the way to the feet and hands. Pay attention to your breathing and allow it to settle lower in the body, and to slow down naturally. When you feel calm and relaxed, rise and begin standing practice, followed by your t'ai chi form.

Taoist Breathing

The connection between breath, vital energy and consciousness is recognized by all the ancient spiritual traditions, and each has practices that work with the breath to achieve energetic balance and states of greater awareness. The expression "breath is life" is not an exaggeration: fail to take your next breath, and your life will soon end. Breathe well, and you will greatly enhance your life – physically, energetically and mentally.

Breathing is essential on a physical level, but its energetic meaning is also very profound – you gather and release energy with every breath in and out.

The state of your internal energy is instantly reflected in your breath: any emotion, such as anger, shock or sadness, immediately affects its quality. Conversely, the way you breathe has an immediate effect on your mental and emotional state. Try breathing rapidly and shallowly (from the chest) for a few moments, as if frightened or angry, then let your breath relax again and become slower and deeper (from the belly). Observe any changes in your mental and/or emotional state. This direct link between the physical breath, your chi and your mind is extremely useful in self-development practice. Breathing work is by far the single most powerful practice you can do.

In the Taoist tradition the breath is never held. Instead, absolute relaxation of the breath is cultivated, allowing it to become progressively smoother in its transition from yin

(breathing in) to yang (breathing out) and back again. The breath is encouraged to drop to the lower tantien, making it the centre of your breathing. When this happens, your lower tantien is awakened and energized and your awareness enters it. This helps to cultivate mental stillness. The same approach exists in other traditions; there is a saying in Zen Buddhism that there is a "Buddha in your belly".

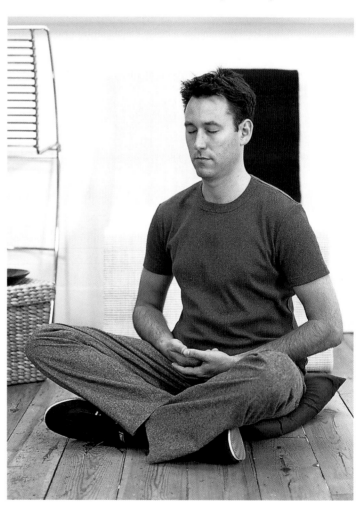

Above When sitting in a chair for breathing practice, align your limbs with your side channels. Check that your spine is straight, without being tense, your head "suspended", the occiput open. Relax your chest and belly, tongue gently touching your palate. Place your hands palms down on your knees, or rest them in your lap.

Above If you are comfortable sitting cross-legged on the floor, make sure your posture is symmetrical to left and right. Sit on a cushion so that your hips are slightly raised, and make sure your midriff and solar plexus area remains open, not collapsed. Your chest and belly must remain totally relaxed to allow your breath to drop.

BREATHING PRACTICE

Follow your breath in through your nose and down to the top of your throat. Be aware of all the sensations it generates, from the physical, to the energetic, to the emotional. As you breathe out, follow your breath back along this pathway, and relax and let go of everything you feel, allowing your energy to release fully. Continue breathing along this pathway until you feel your breath dropping lower, into your throat.

Let your breathing become progressively more relaxed and continuous (from in to out, without holding or stopping), following the breath as it naturally drops through the centreline of your body. Continue to be aware of your internal sensations on each in-breath, and relax and let go of whatever you feel with every out-breath. It may take several weeks of daily practice to get your breathing to relax sufficiently to enter your lower tantien. Do not force the pace – it will only increase your level of internal tension, and is counterproductive. As you continue breathing you will find that your breath naturally becomes longer and slower, allowing the mind to relax and become still. Encourage this process, but without forcing yourself to breathe slowly.

Eventually, you will feel that your lower tantien fills and empties with every in- and out-breath, and that you are no longer breathing from your chest. As the tantien fills, your

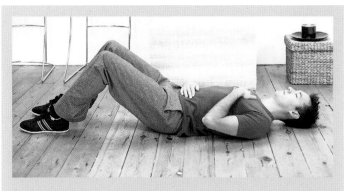

Breathing practice lying down
If you prefer to do the breathing sequence lying down, place your hands on your chest and tantien, and allow your body to sink deeper into the floor with every out-breath.

breath (and chi) will "overflow" to energize the whole pelvic area, and then the organs and spine. If you feel this process happening, you can lead your breath to different parts of your body, but do not push it. Remember that as much as you breathe in and energize, you also relax and let go on the out-breath. If you feel that you are breathing through your legs or feet, without effort, simply allow it to happen (this forms part of the more advanced process of "reverse breathing" alluded to in the Tao Te Ching: "The Wise Man breathes through his heels"). Never deliberately push your breath below your lower tantien as this can cause problems with your sexual energy. Follow the exercises, both on your own and with a partner holding the areas indicated and giving you verbal feedback.

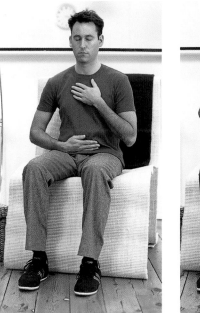 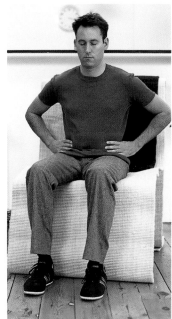

1 Place one palm on your chest and one over your tantien to make you aware of the relative proportions of your breath in your upper and lower body. Relax your chest and belly, allowing your breath to sink. Then move your hands to just above your pelvic bone. Feel the front and sides of your abdomen – the tantien area – fill and empty with your breath.

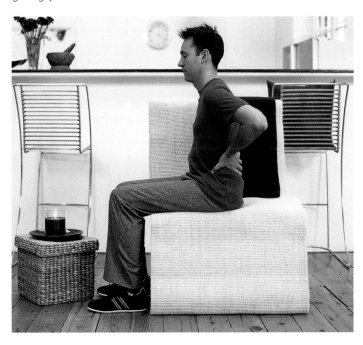

2 Next place your hands near your kidneys, to feel the back of your abdominal area expand and release with your breath. Do not force your breath into your kidney area – be gentle. Try to achieve equal movement and relaxation on the left and right sides of your body.

Standing Practice

The purpose of this is to start feeling and releasing blockages and misalignments in your body, and to activate the downward, yin flow of energy within you, from heaven to earth. This assists in the dissolving of blockages as well as stilling the mind.

Standing practice is the foundation stone of the internal arts, essential to releasing blockage and building power. Ideally, you should stand for at least 10 minutes every day. It is not unusual for dedicated practitioners to stand for over an hour in one session, but you should build up your practice time very gradually.

TUCKING THE TAILBONE

The following pages detail the important body alignments of t'ai chi, and one of the major emphases is on "tucking" the tailbone. It is easy to misunderstand this principle. It does not mean that you should push or force your pelvis down and under, as this just creates tension in the very area that you are seeking to release. It means allowing the back of the pelvis to drop under its own weight. This requires you to relax your abdominal muscles, letting the front of the pelvis "hollow". At first this will result in a very small physical movement. However, it allows the sacrum and lower back to release, and over time the pelvis will drop considerably when allowed to do so. The end result is that the tailbone will naturally curve under the pelvic area, with a feeling as if it is threading through the back of the knees. When this process is complete, your spinal energy will connect from the tailbone through the back of the knees and the ankles, and through the Bubbling Well point on the foot, where it will join with the energy of the earth. The tailbone feels as if it is penetrating the foot. This is known as "rooting".

T'AI CHI MOVEMENT

The key principles in moving in a t'ai chi way are circularity and balance. Circularity means both moving the limbs in circles and curves – rather than in straight lines – and also moving continuously, flowing from yin to yang and back again without stops or gaps in the movement. This allows your chi to start flowing and continue flowing smoothly. The t'ai chi classics state: "From posture to posture the internal energy should be continuous and unbroken." This is one of the defining characteristics of t'ai chi.

MAKING PROGRESS

Many t'ai chi practitioners find that they go through periods of apparently little progress in their practice, followed by sudden "leaps". You may find this is the case with you. The "less rewarding" phases are actually very important, as it is during these times that you are integrating t'ai chi principles and your system is processing the new information. The leaps happen when the process of integration is complete. It is best to be neither disheartened by the less exciting periods of practice nor too triumphant or over-excited by any sudden progress. Learning t'ai chi is a cyclical process, with one phase following another. Regular, relaxed practice is the best route to progress.

PREPARING YOUR STANCE

After preparing for standing practice by lying down and releasing the nervous system, you are ready to start the standing posture. Stand with your weight equally distributed on both feet. Your chest and belly should remain relaxed at all times, as this allows your chi to drop down the yin channels at the front of your body. It will then naturally rise up the yang channels in the back of the body. "Sink the chest to raise the back" is the phrase that expresses this. A sense of "melting" down the front of your body (including your face) is ideal. Pay special attention to the occiput at the base of your skull: gently draw your chin back and slightly downwards, as if you were tipping the brim of a hat. This opens the energy gate at the occiput. Keep space in your armpits – as if you had a golf ball under each one.

A partner should check you are not leaning back with your upper body, which is very common in beginners. Allow them to correct you, even if it makes you feel as if you are falling forwards (this feeling will pass). Your feet should be parallel even if it feels strange at first – this opens your sacrum. Always keep space in your perineum (between your legs). Feel as if your tailbone threads through the back of your knees, causing them to bend as you allow the back of your pelvis to drop. Feel as if you are sitting into your legs.

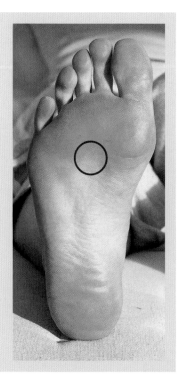

The Bubbling Well
Shown here by the red circle is the Bubbling Well point in the foot. You can find this point by curling your toes forward. The hollow that appears in the location marked is the Bubbling Well.

The Five Points
The five points are: the Bubbling Well in both feet, the laogung point in the centre of both palms, and the baihui point at the crown of the head. Maintain full awareness of these points during chi gung and t'ai chi practice to fully circulate chi.

Standing Posture

These illustrations show the major body alignments for standing practice and t'ai chi. This posture is called wu chi ("total emptiness"). Follow the annotations and, if possible, have a partner check your posture.

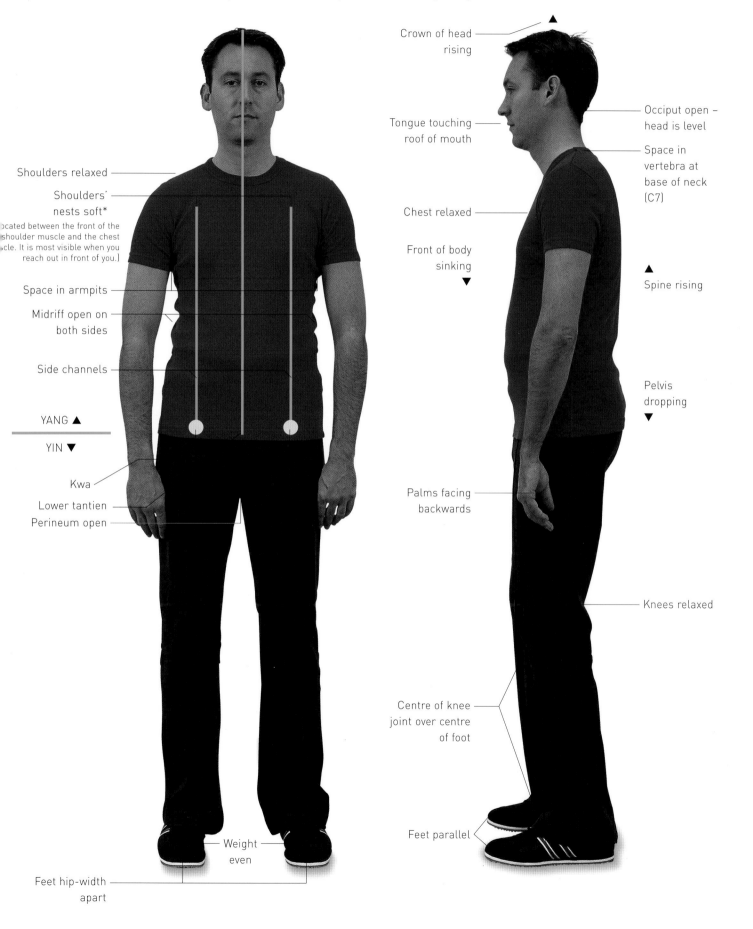

Shoulders relaxed

Shoulders' nests soft*

located between the front of the shoulder muscle and the chest muscle. It is most visible when you reach out in front of you.)

Space in armpits

Midriff open on both sides

Side channels

YANG ▲

YIN ▼

Kwa

Lower tantien

Perineum open

Weight even

Feet hip-width apart

Crown of head rising

Tongue touching roof of mouth

Chest relaxed

Front of body sinking ▼

Occiput open – head is level

Space in vertebra at base of neck (C7)

▲ Spine rising

Pelvis dropping ▼

Palms facing backwards

Knees relaxed

Centre of knee joint over centre of foot

Feet parallel

Kwa Squat and Tuck

The kwa is a key area in t'ai chi and all the Taoist internal arts. In anatomical terms,
it is known as the inguinal fold, located at the front of the pelvis. It is easy to find, as
it is the area that folds when you sit.

A relaxed kwa allows for strong chi flow through that area, for the efficient pumping of the fluids of the body, especially blood and lymph, and for the release of tension throughout the pelvis, especially the sacrum. As a general principle, the front of the body governs the back of the body – it is essential that you release the front of your body if you wish to release the back of your body. To find your kwa, first find your hip bones at the front of your pelvis. Now move inwards and downwards with both hands until your fingers fall into a softer area at either side of the front of your groin. This area will naturally fold as you squat or sit.

Do the following exercise several times until you gain a greater sense of blood and chi flow through your legs, and you can feel your kwa softening. When leaning forward, keep your spine straight, from tailbone to crown of head, along the angle of incline. Do not take your front knee beyond your front toes as this may strain the knee joint. If you find the heel of your rear foot rises, reposition your rear foot closer to the front foot (that is, shorten your stance). Repeat the forward squat and tuck on one side, then change legs and do an equal number on the other side.

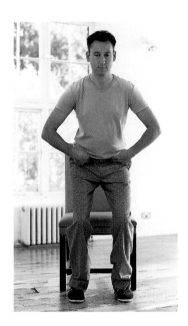

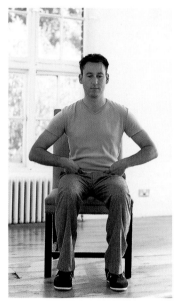

1 Standing in front of a chair, use your fingers to find the kwa as you lower into a squat. Relax deeply into that place.

2 Let yourself fall gently into the chair, simply by relaxing your kwa.

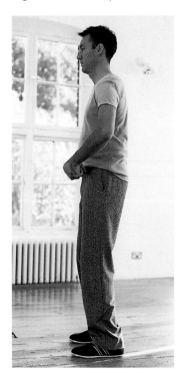

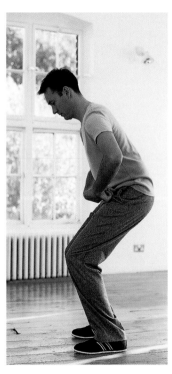

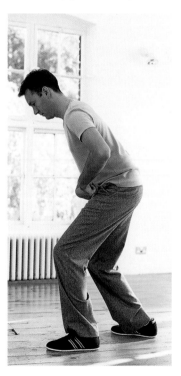

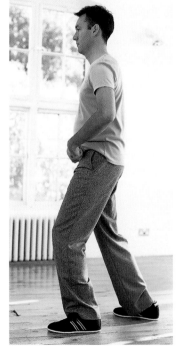

3 Continue your kwa squats without a chair, allowing your upper body to lean forward naturally as you descend. Don't squat too low. Keep your spine straight, from tailbone to crown of head, along the angle of incline. Stand up again and repeat.

4 Take a step forward, keeping your feet the same width apart as in standing practice. With all your weight on your front leg, squat into your kwa. Let your left and right kwa fold equally. Make sure you allow your rear leg to bend, and note that the angle of your spine and the angle of your lower rear leg are the same. Keeping all your weight on your front leg, stand up, opening your kwa and bringing your pelvis forward.

Weight Transfer

This exercise will help you develop the smooth transfer of your body weight from one leg to the other, while remaining "rooted", or connected with the ground. Transfer your weight as if you were pouring water continuously from one bottle into another.

When you transfer your weight smoothly, retaining this connection, it switches the up/down flows of chi to the opposite side of the body. Chi drops through the weighted leg into the ground and rises up the unweighted leg from the ground. Feel as if your weighted leg pushes you on to your unweighted leg.

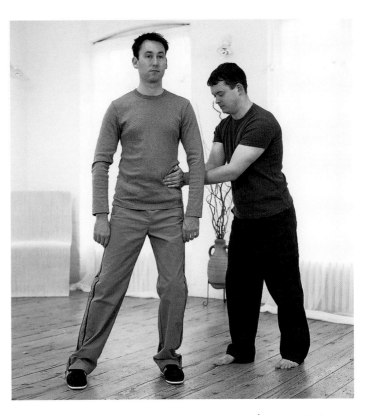

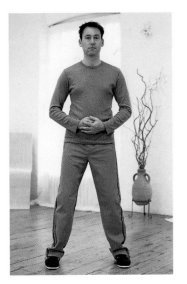 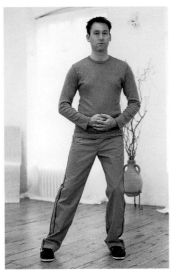

1 Start in an equally weighted position with your feet about 1½ shoulder-widths apart. Transfer your weight smoothly from the right side to the left, maintaining the connection from your spine to the ground, and moving that connection to the left until it passes fully through your left leg. You have now transferred your "root" to your left leg. Make sure your left hip joint doesn't "pop out" to the side. Now transfer your weight back to the centre, and then to your right leg.

2 Ask your partner to apply steady resistance (making their body rigid as if it were a piece of wood) to the side of your hip as you transfer your weight. Notice how you need to stay "dropped" through your legs (rooted) in order to move them without effort.

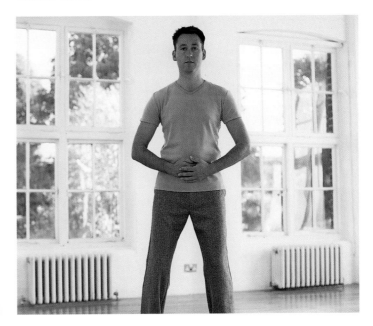

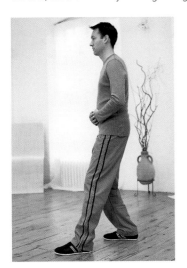 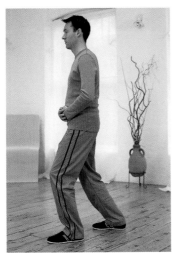

3 Step forward and stand with your weight on your back leg. Keeping your spine upright and your head suspended, transfer your weight smoothly to your front leg. Feel your energetic "root" transferring from your back leg to your front leg.

4 Ask your partner to apply resistance at the front of your hips, and repeat, concentrating on smoothness and relaxing into your legs. Now practise shifting your weight alternately backwards and forwards. Change legs and repeat.

Unifying

The exercises shown here help you unify your upper and lower body. The key to this is your spine – every part of your body should feel as if it is connected to it. When you unify your body your chi will also become unified and flow smoothly and strongly.

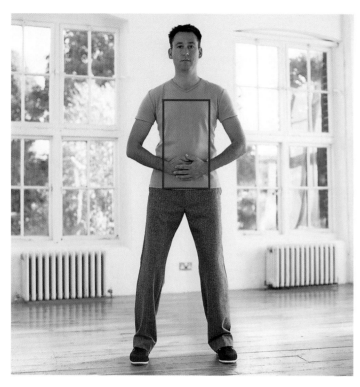

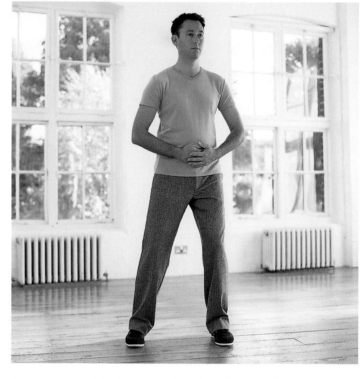

1 The "four points" (the shoulder's nest and kwa on each side) should always be linked as if they form a rectangle – you should not allow this shape to twist or distort. This means turning your spine as a unit along its length without twisting it.

2 Turn to one side, then the other, keeping your four points linked. Feel as if the movement originates in your lower tantien and your spine turns as a unit. Keep your spine vertical, without tilting to one side or the other.

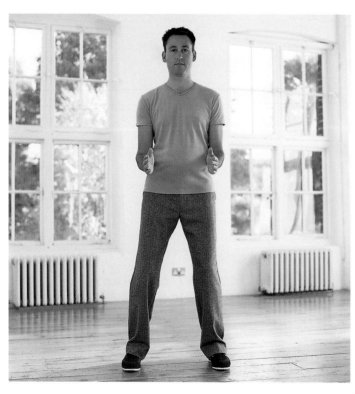

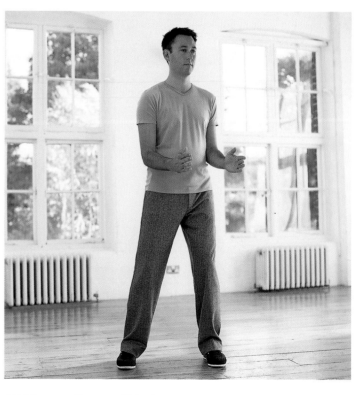

3 Lock your elbows at your sides, your hands pointing forward, feeling the connection between your upper and lower body.

4 With your elbows still locked at your sides, turn to the left. Turn back to the centre and then to the right.

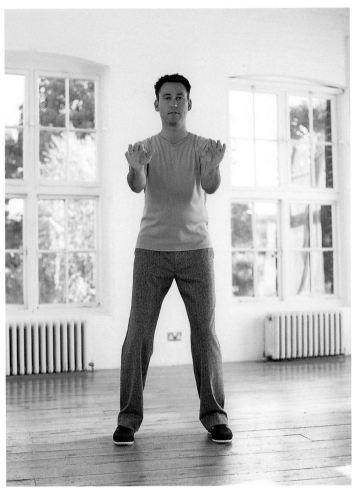

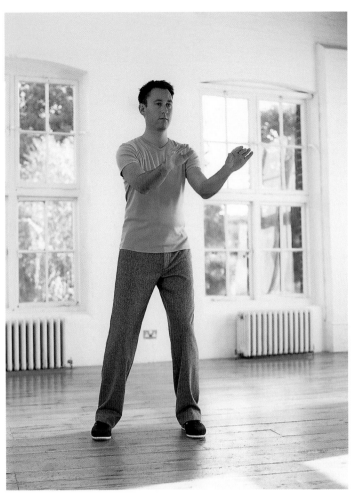

5 Hold your arms out in front of you, elbow tips pointing at the floor and palms down. This part of the exercise will help you develop the ability to link your arms to your spine, helping your chi flow smoothly from your tantien to your fingertips.

6 Turn to the left, keeping your arms linked to your spine, feeling that your spine is turning and your arms are simply attached. The movement should originate in the spine and not in the arms. Turn back to the centre and then to the right.

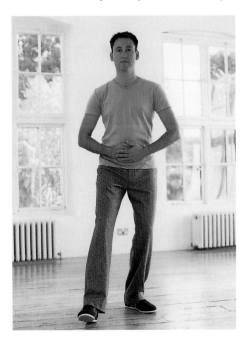

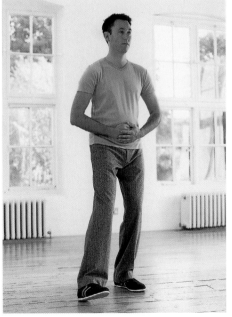

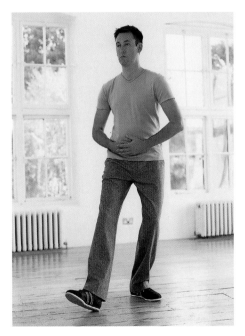

7 Take a step forward, keeping all your weight on your back leg, with the heel of your front foot resting on the floor, then turn in the direction of your weighted leg, folding into the kwa on that side. Let your unweighted leg turn as well, feeling the connection to your spine. Your tantien and spine are the origin of the movement, and your upper and lower torso do not twist in relation to one another. Keep your weighted knee fixed.

8 Turn 45 degrees from the centre in the opposite direction. Keep your weighted knee still, and don't let it twist. Turn back into your weighted kwa again, and repeat. Then change legs, and continue.

Stepping

When a cat steps, it carefully places a paw in front of it, not committing its weight until ready, then rolls through the paw surface from back to front. T'ai chi stepping is similar. The same principle applies whether you are stepping forward or back.

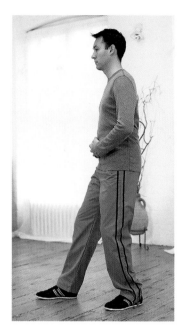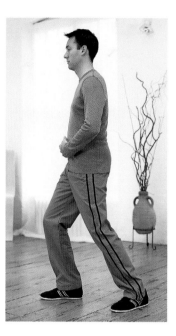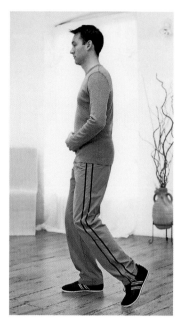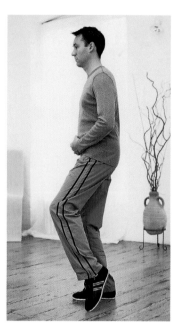

1 Start with your weight on your back leg. Shift 100% of your weight forward, transferring your root to your front leg, while maintaining an upright spine and proper alignments. As you move, try to maintain a level height. Look straight ahead and not downwards.

2 Peel your back foot off the ground and bring it level with your front foot. Have a sense of your kwa closing and "sucking" your back leg in and forward to this point.

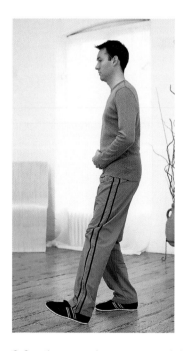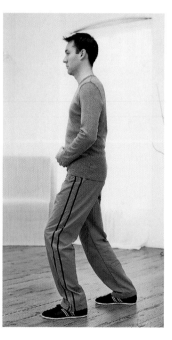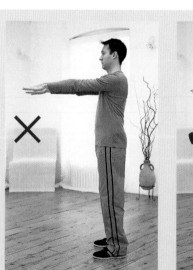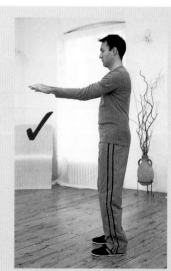

3 Continue moving your unweighted foot forward and place your heel on the ground in front of you, without shifting your weight to it. Have a sense of your kwa opening and "spitting out" your front leg to bring it forward. Transfer your weight to your front foot, from your heel to the ball of your foot. Repeat with your other leg and continue stepping forward, alternating sides.

The Comfort Zone

Overextending the arms locks the joints and blocks the flow of chi, so approximately 30 per cent bend is retained in the extended arms, keeping within the comfort zone. The same applies to the legs. None of your joints should be locked open or completely closed at any time in t'ai chi or chi gung practice. When bringing your arms in towards your body, fold your joints to a maximum of only 70 per cent.

Raising the Arms

This sequence shows how to raise your arms during t'ai chi and chi gung practice.
Think of your arm as a lever, with your shoulder joint as the pivot and your
shoulder blade as a counterweight.

As your arm rises, your shoulder stays relaxed, not rising at all, and your shoulder blade drops down your back. Over time, this helps to release your shoulder blades, and thus your entire upper back and neck area. Keep a sense of your elbows being heavy, as if weighted down, throughout your practice. Raise your arms only as far as you can while keeping your shoulders relaxed and a sense of your shoulder blades dropping.

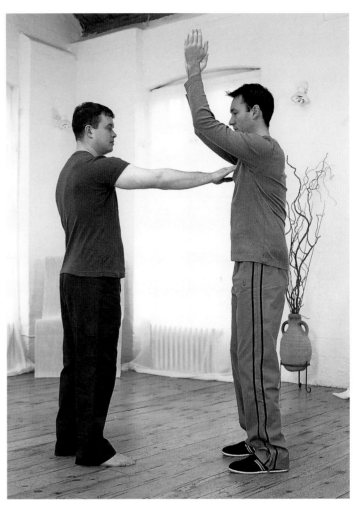

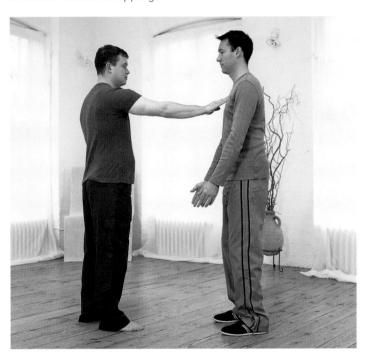

1 Start raising your arms with a partner touching your chest at the sternum (breastbone), to ensure that you do not raise your chest at any point during the exercise.

2 Relax the front of your body as your arms rise, ideally feeling that your chest and belly sink more the higher your arms go. A sense of dropping down through your side channels is ideal.

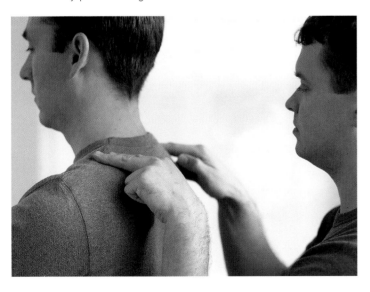

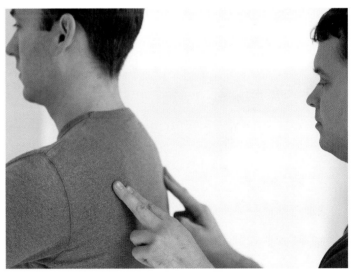

3 Raise your arms again with your partner touching your trapezius muscle, to ensure you do not lift your shoulders.

4 Raise your arms again with your partner touching the centre of each shoulder blade, to help you drop them down your back.

Relaxing and Releasing

T'ai chi is about learning to relax your body, energy and mind, and release tensions and blockages on all those levels. The techniques that follow help you with that process and prepare you for your t'ai chi form practice. You can continue to work with these exercises as secondary methods alongside your form practice. Remember that the most essential principle of t'ai chi is to relax and soften habitual tension, wherever you encounter it.

You can repeat the "washing downwards" exercise as many times as you wish. You may find you encounter and release different blockages with every repetition. If you find you start to shake spontaneously, allow this to happen, without manipulating it. This indicates the partial release of chi blockages and is perfectly normal. When your alignments are correct, it will feel as if your body holds itself up against gravity, with no conscious effort on your part.

WASHING DOWNWARDS

Align your body in the wu chi standing position. Consciously relax the soles of your feet, ideally until you lose any clear sense of where your feet end and where the floor begins. This will allow your chi to release through your feet and into the ground. Then relax your ankles, knees and kwa. Bounce a little on your legs to get a sense of being relaxed and springy in your kwa and your knee and ankle joints. Your lower body, from your tantien down, should feel heavy and sinking (yin). At the same time you should feel as if the crown of your head is floating upwards and your upper body from the tantien up is very light and empty (yang), but without raising your chest. This simultaneous sinking and rising opens your body between your head and your feet. The overall feeling is that you lengthen in opposite directions from your tantien: down through your feet, and up through your crown. Your tantien is the central point. This feeling should be maintained throughout all t'ai chi and chi gung practice. It ensures that your chi becomes full from the top to the bottom of your body. Be aware of the five points of t'ai chi: feet, crown and palms.

Once you feel settled in your posture, take your attention to the crown of your head and, as if you have a sheet of water there, allow it to start dropping through you, washing tension away. Allow it to wash through your arms at the same height as your body. Take this feeling all the way down, through your legs, out of your feet and beneath you, into the ground. Pay special attention along the way to releasing the main energy gates listed earlier. Always take this "washing downwards" process from the crown of your head fully into the ground.

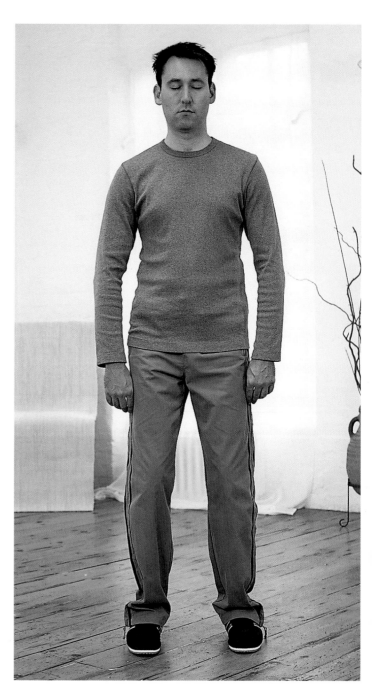

Above As you stand, have a sense of allowing release to occur only if it is ready, rather than expecting set results. This allows for greater relaxation and consequently greater release of blockages.

ARM DROPS

This exercise can be done solo or with a partner. If you are working on your own, raise your arms above your head and let them fall freely. Repeat several times, trying to let go of any tension in your arms as you let them fall.

If you are working with a partner, ask them to hold your arms above your head while you relax them completely. Concentrate on relaxing all the nerves in your arms and shoulders. Your partner can then release your arms, and, if they are relaxed, they will fall freely, swinging and "bouncing" at the bottom of their swing. If they do not, you are holding tension in them, so repeat until you release all residual tension in your arms.

DROPPING THE PELVIS

This exercise helps you develop a sense of letting go of your lower back and sacrum, to allow your pelvis to drop. Stand facing a wall with your toes about 30cm (12in) from it, and arms reaching upwards, palms on the wall. Progressively allow your pelvis to drop, and feel your spine lengthening downwards from the base of your neck, and the spaces between your vertebrae increasing. Return to your "normal" pelvic position and repeat. Get your partner to place a hand on your sacrum (at the back of the pelvis), to focus your awareness and encourage relaxation and dropping.

Below Dropping the pelvis is a core part of getting your spine to connect energetically with the earth.

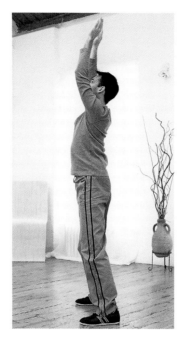
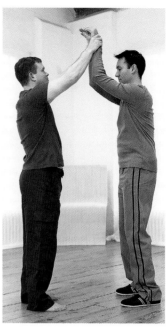

Above Raise your arms above your head and then let them fall as freely as you can.

Above Try to let go of your arms completely so that they fall immediately when released.

SHOULDER'S NEST

Tension in your shoulder's nest locks tension into your upper back. Ask your partner to place two fingers in your shoulder's nest as they gently draw your arm towards them. Try to relax your shoulder's nest to allow their fingers to sink into the area, without your partner applying any pressure. This will result in your shoulder (including the shoulder blade) releasing forwards and moving off your back. Change arms and repeat.

Below Hollowing the shoulder's nest allows your back to open, giving your lungs more space and helping chi flow through the arms.

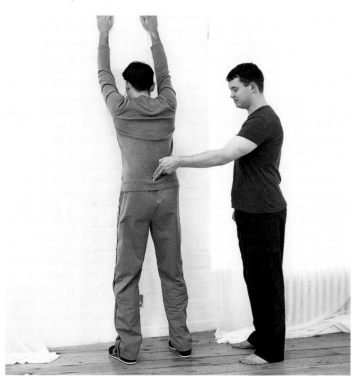

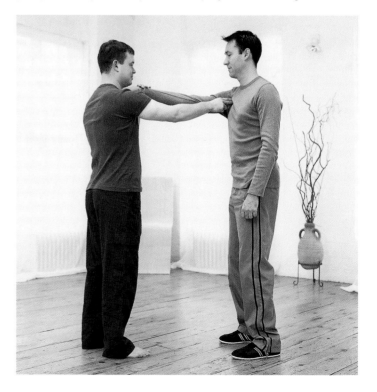

DRAWING THE ARMS

Stand with your back flat against a wall and have your partner hold both your arms at the wrists, supporting the weight of your arms. They should then very gently draw your arms equally towards them, opening your back and releasing your shoulders. When they start to encounter resistance, they should hold that position and very softly jiggle your arms (like jiggling a length of rope), until they sense your nervous system relax. They can then draw your arms out a little further, until your nerves start to tense again. Go through several cycles of drawing out and releasing, each time releasing your back a little more.

Eventually this releasing will extend through the length of your back, from your shoulder blades to your buttocks. See the arrows for the direction of release of your body's tissues.

SQUATS

Standing, raise your arms above your head. Then squat into your kwa, allowing the back of your spine to relax and curve open as you go. Finish with your hands behind your feet as shown, and tailbone curved slightly under your pelvis. This movement releases the back of your body and exercises your kwa fold.

Now open the front of your body, generating the movement from your kwa. As you raise yourself upright, raise your arms, palms facing out, until you are fully upright, with your hands above you. Feel the opening and stretching running from your toes to your fingertips (along

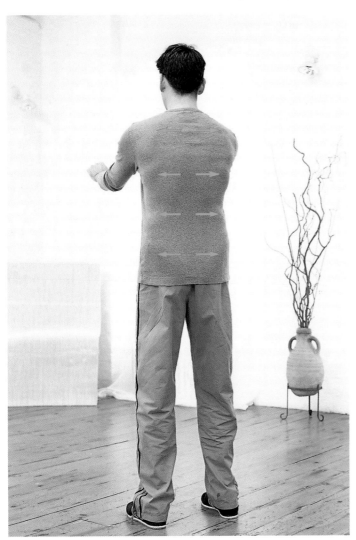

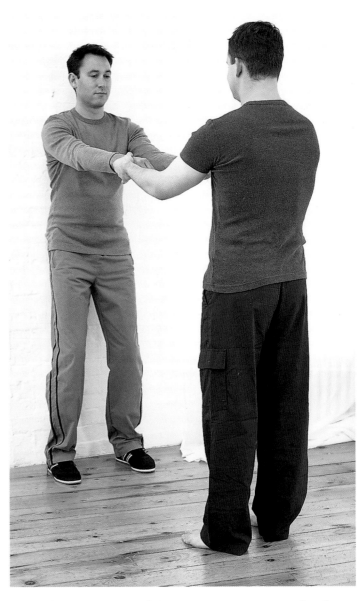

Above The lengthening of the body's tissues horizontally is known as "wrapping". This "wrapping" or spreading can extend the entire length of the body, to include the legs and feet. It moves chi from the back of the body to the front, and vice versa (wrapping front to back).

Above Drawing the arms. Relax your nervous system so that the fascia of your back can release and wrap forwards. Your partner can actively help you relax your nerves and expand your back, while you remain relaxed and passive, just letting it happen.

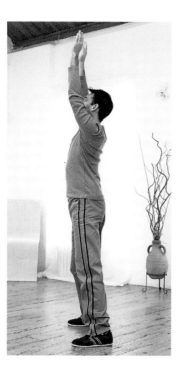

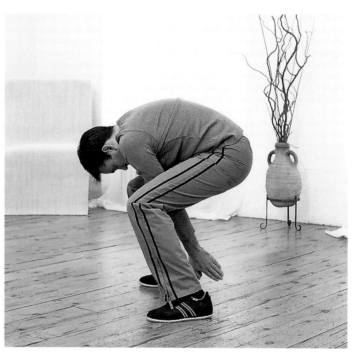

Right and far right Squats. These open the front of the body from the tips of the toes to the fingertips. Keep the chest and belly relaxed as you do this, if possible opening the body in a wavelike motion from the feet to the fingers. Start with your hands together, above your head, then lean forwards and squat into the kwa. Only go as low as you feel comfortable, without putting any strain on your knees. Relax and let your head drop as you bend.

your inner arms). Do not arch your spine more than a minimal amount. This movement releases the front of your body and your spine and opens your kwa. Relaxing the back of your body, squat again and repeat.

RELEASING THE HIPS

Lying on your back, bring your knees up and hold them in the palms of your hands. Relax your hip joints and legs, and using your hands – not your legs – to do the work, make circles with your knees, first towards each other, and then in the reverse direction. Allow this circular motion to move into your hip joints and sacrum, releasing them. During this exercise you may find that similar circling and releasing occurs spontaneously in your shoulders.

DRAWING THE LEGS

Have your partner raise one of your legs by the foot, and perform the drawing out/jiggling action they did with your arms, as if wiggling a rope to make a wave travel through it. This is to lengthen the tissues of your leg, hip and lower back, and release binding and contraction in these areas. They should not pull hard or jiggle forcefully. Ideally, this should create a wavelike motion along the length of your leg. After releasing one leg, repeat with the other. If your partner can support the weight of both legs, they can hold your feet parallel, jiggling them at the same time in a horizontal motion to get a wavelike releasing to travel from your feet through your legs and hips, up your spine, to your head. This can be extremely relaxing if done gently and well.

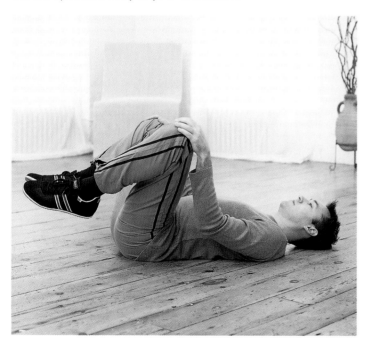

Above Hip joints tend to become extremely stiff and blocked as they bear the entire body's weight. Circling your hips can help release these joints, allowing you deeper access while doing t'ai chi form.

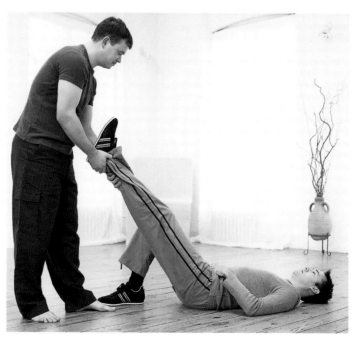

Above When working with the legs, be very gentle, as they connect directly into the sacrum and spine. No force should ever be used while jiggling and releasing the legs with a partner.

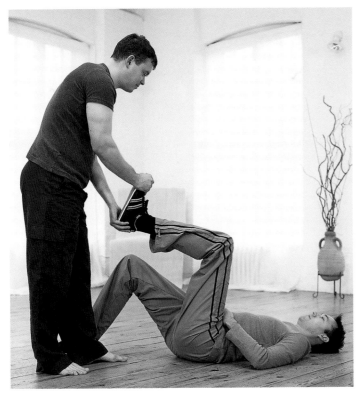

Above With misaligned leg joints, the line of force from walking and running will not pass through smoothly and over time joint damage will occur. Correct joint alignments will prevent this happening.

SPRING IN THE LEGS

Have your partner raise one of your legs by the foot, and align the centre of your foot with the centre of your ankle joint, the centre of your knee joint and the centre of your hip joint. They should then test the alignment by gently pushing along the axis of your joints while you gently push back. If the alignments are correct, there will be an easy springiness in

Right and Far right Circling hands reflects the way t'ai chi involves making circles throughout the form. These circles start on a more external level, and then they become internalized, until you are making circles at increasingly deep levels within your body, and within your energy. This can have the effect of eliminating linear, "stuck" patterns in your energy and also in your mental processes, helping you to adapt to changing circumstances with an easy flow.

all the joints, which will rebound towards your partner once compressed. If incorrect, your joints will feel "dead", and you will feel that it requires some effort to push back at your partner. When you have achieved the correct alignment, remember how it feels so you can replicate it for yourself while doing t'ai chi (you can bounce on your legs while standing or doing t'ai chi in order to check this).

CIRCLES

Standing, interlock your fingers and circle your thumbs around one another in both directions. Then position one hand close to you and one further away, but both on the centreline of your body, palms facing you. Circle your hands around each other vertically, trying to make as perfect a circle as you can. Once you are comfortable with this, vary the diameter of your circles, from very small (fingers almost touching) to very large (arms' length). Then reverse the direction. Over time, try to make this movement originate from nearer your body (fingers to wrists to elbows to shoulder joints) until you are circling from your shoulders.

Next, place the palm of one hand over the back of the other hand and hold them out horizontally in front of you. Make circles in the horizontal plane, keeping the centre of the circles on your centreline (so your hands go to the left and right sides of your body and towards and away from you). Circle in both directions. Over time, bring the circles up into – and from – your shoulder blades.

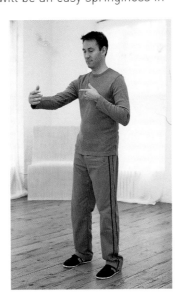

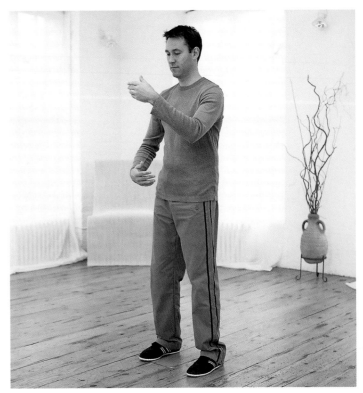

SWING

This exercise releases your lower back and pelvic area, as well as energizing the lower organs (the area known as the lower jiao). Pay special attention to the instructions on leg and hip alignments while moving and turning, as these apply directly to both the Cloud Hands chi gung exercise and t'ai chi form practice.

Stand with your feet parallel, 1½ shoulder-widths apart, and transfer your weight from side to side maintaining all the principles learned so far. Build up a regular, steady rhythm. Once this is well established, turn your centre (maintaining your "four points") to your weighted side as you shift your weight. Fold into your weighted kwa, as shown in the unifying exercises. As you turn, keep both knees steady, facing forward at all times – have a partner gently hold each kneecap, to assist in this. Never twist your knee joints or you may injure them. Leave your arms as relaxed as in the arm drop exercise; as you release your body and your motion becomes smoother, they will naturally swing towards and away from your body, gathering and releasing energy as they do so. Your weight shift should power the entire movement. Keep your head suspended and allow your pelvis to drop, letting tension release from your spine.

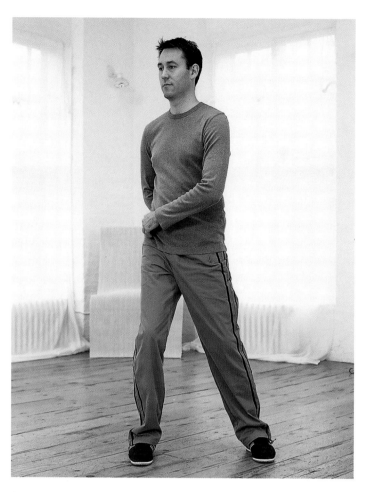

Above Swinging to the right. Note the folding into the weighted kwa, the spine turning as a unit, keeping the four points together. The head is suspended and the spine upright but relaxed.

Below Swinging to the left. As your arms relax and swing more freely you can allow them to tap your body gently as they come in. Make sure you keep your weighted knee still and do not twist it.

Below Working with a partner to ensure there is no twisting in the knees. By keeping the knees fixed and simultaneously turning to the side, the leg tissues are released by spiralling around the leg bones.

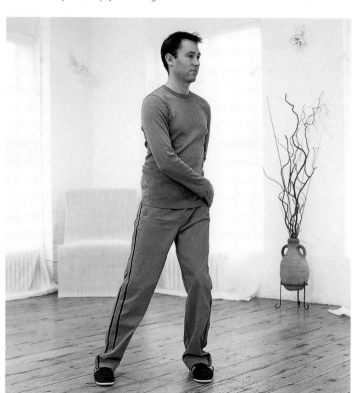

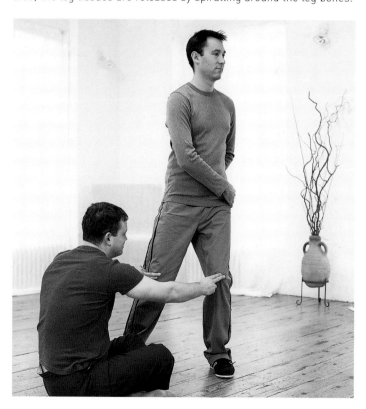

Cloud Hands

This complete chi gung exercise contains many key elements of Taoist nei gung, which are also fundamental to t'ai chi. It uses the weight shifting, turning and spiralling actions of t'ai chi, and teaches you how to spiral your arms in opposite directions simultaneously. It incorporates the key principles of t'ai chi, and therefore it is traditionally said that if you can do Cloud Hands well, then you can do t'ai chi well.

Cloud Hands works the upward and downward flows of energy in your body (on opposite sides), as well as the outward and inward flows from periphery to centre, and from centre to periphery. It activates spiralling energy in your body and releases your body through twistings of your tissues and pulsings of the joints and spaces of your body. It also activates the yin and yang meridians of your body, and unifies physical and chi movement into an integral whole. The way you shift weight, turn and connect your arms to your entire body through your spine is exactly the same as in t'ai chi. Cloud Hands embodies the essence of t'ai chi, and by practising it you will gain many of the benefits of t'ai chi practice in a very simple and easily learned form.

WHOLE BODY

During Cloud Hands your weight shift, turn and arm spiralling should be proportional: for example, at 20 per cent of your shift to one side, you will have turned through 20 per cent of your range of movement to that side, and will have spiralled your arms 20 per cent of their range. Make your movements flowing and continuous from one side to the other, and do not exceed your comfort zone of 70 per cent of your maximum range of movement. You are bringing energy up the unweighted side of your body to the fingertips of your raised hand, and dropping it down the weighted side, and down through the bottom palm. Turn your hands proportionately to the amount you raise and lower them.

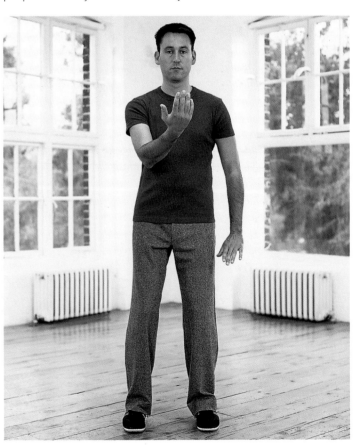

1 Standing evenly weighted, hold your hands palms facing each other as shown here. You will move both arms simultaneously.

2 Bring your right hand up and out until your palm is facing your mouth. Lower your left hand until it is facing palm down.

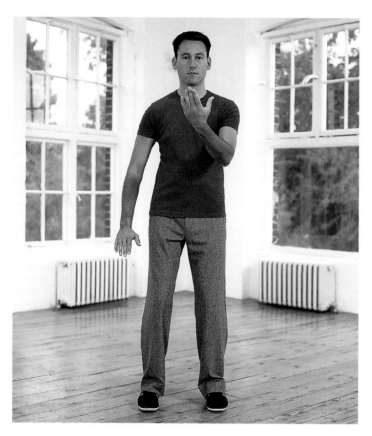

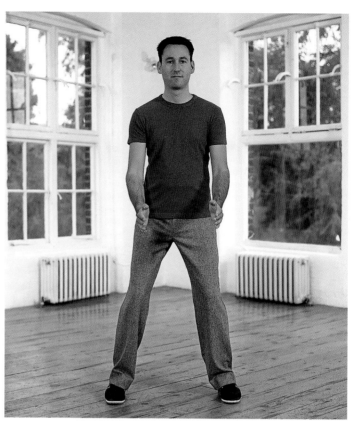

3 Reverse your movement to return to the starting point, and then repeat with the arms moving in the opposite direction (left rises and right drops).

4 Standing with your feet about 1½ shoulder-widths apart, and parallel, start with your hands in the same position as before, in front of your lower tantien.

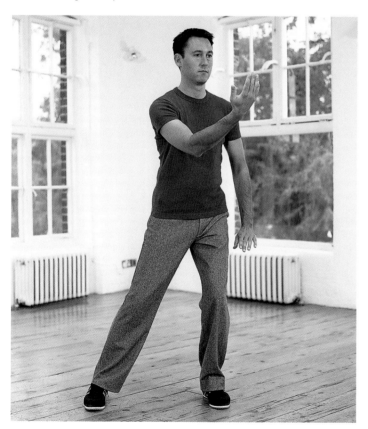

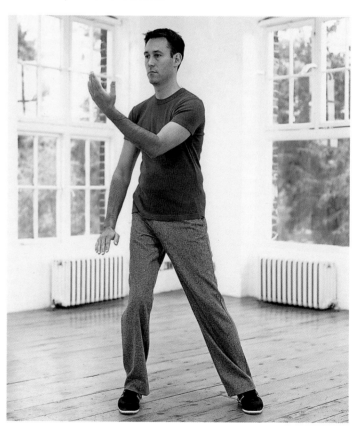

5 Transfer your weight to the left, and turn your centre to the left (folding into your left kwa). Remember to apply the t'ai chi movement principles that you have learned. As you shift your weight and turn, spiral your arms exactly as in the previous exercise. Do not bring your upper arm past your centreline.

6 Start shifting and turning back to the centre, spiralling your arms in reverse. When you return to the centre, start shifting and turning to the right, simultaneously spiralling your left arm upwards and your right arm downwards. Once you are fully shifted and turned, repeat to the other side.

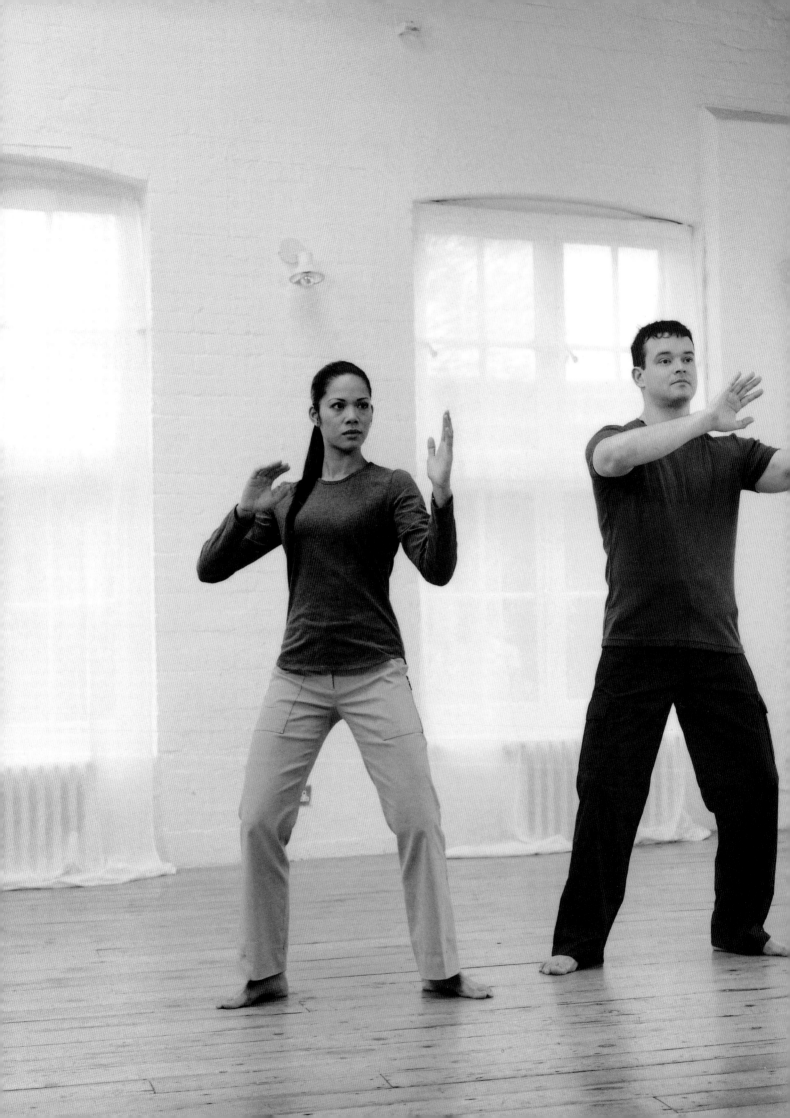

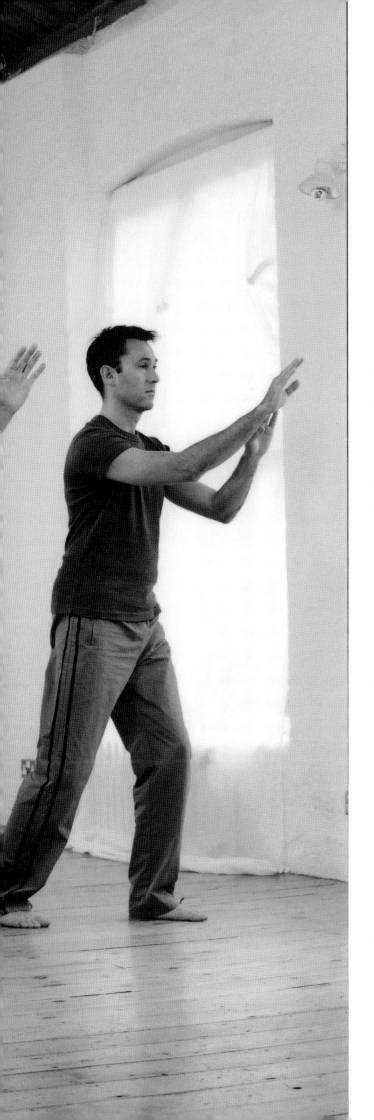

The Wu Style Short Form

This chapter contains a full Wu style t'ai chi short form, clearly illustrated and explained. The main practice in t'ai chi consists of a set, or form, of flowing movements. Each posture in the form leads into the next and each has a different function. The exact functions of each movement are best learned directly from a teacher, but by following the instructions here, and maintaining t'ai chi principles of body alignment and movement, you will start to gain the benefits of t'ai chi practice. Because the essence of t'ai chi is embodied in its principles, almost any physical movement could be adapted to become a "t'ai chi" movement. However, it is also inherently a martial art, so its postures relate to specific fighting techniques. The form is structured in such a way that these postures flow one into another to maximize the release of the body and the smooth flow of chi, as well as the gathering and releasing of chi.

Introducing the Form

The Wu style short form contains many of the postures of the long form and offers most of its benefits, but it is far easier to learn and much quicker to perform, and requires much less space. This makes the short form highly suitable not only for beginners but also for anyone with limited time and practice space. The short form can be extended by being practised back-to-back, flowing seamlessly from one form repetition into the next.

T'ai chi forms are generally divided into short and long forms. Long forms have certain advantages and also certain disadvantages, such as taking a long time to learn and requiring more time and space to practise.

BREATHING AND RELEASING
As you proceed through the form, relax your breathing. Do not impose a set pattern of in-/out-breaths on your movement. If you find that you naturally breathe in or out on certain moves that is fine, but it is very important that you allow this to occur automatically. This is because t'ai chi form practice causes release of emotional tension, and this happens primarily through the breath, as a vibration or charge within it. If you relax your breathing, the releases will occur naturally, but if you impose a pattern on your breathing, you may block releases of emotional energy.

EMPTY AND FULL
In the Wu style of t'ai chi, many postures involve gently touching the radial (thumb side) pulse of one wrist with the fingers of the other hand. This is visibly different to other styles. The reason for doing it is to make a connection with the energy of your internal organs, allowing you to release any blockages.

The yin/yang concept of "empty/full" is central to t'ai chi, and applies to the arms and legs as well as the left and right sides of the body. One hand/arm is full while the other is empty. The hand touching your pulse is empty, while the other is full. The empty hand/arm is supplying chi energy to the full. In relation to your legs, your full leg bears your weight and allows chi to drop down through it into the ground. Your empty leg is unweighted but still in contact with the ground. It is through the empty leg that chi rises from the ground, up through your body and out of your arms. Always keep your unweighted heel on the ground.

When moving outwards (releasing energy), allow your chi to release fully through your hands and fingers into the space outside you, but without "pushing out" mentally. This will help ensure that you eliminate chi stagnation from your system. Keep your eyes relaxed at all times – again, not "pushing out" through them (which causes tension), but keeping them open so that your awareness is present both within you and in the space outside you.

At the end of your form practice, as you return to wu chi standing, feel that you are gathering chi from all parts of your body into your tantien. Allow any sense of agitation or excitement in your energy to settle down, until your chi feels calm and still. Then have a sense of condensing and storing that energy in your tantien. When you feel you cannot store any more, circulate whatever chi is not stored, throughout your body, to energize yourself fully.

Below An outward-moving t'ai chi form posture. Chi energy is circulated fully from the feet to the fingertips and the crown of the head. The gaze is relaxed and directed outwards.

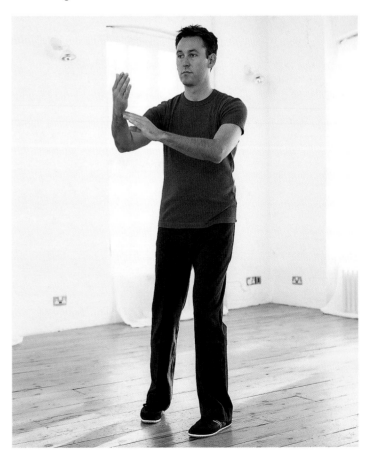

How to Follow the Steps

The form is shown here from beginning to end, in sequence. The main pictures show the movements from a consistent angle to make it easier for you to understand in which direction you should be facing at any given point. Where the position of the arms and/or legs is obscured, for example by a turn, refer to the smaller images in the Alternative View boxes, which clearly show the side of the body hidden in the main image.

The most important thing to remember when following the steps is that t'ai chi is a movement practice, and that the pictures show only set points along a continuum of movement. Some of these points are the "final" positions of the postures, others are transitional points. However, even the "final" positions are in themselves transitions into the next posture: in t'ai chi you never stop, but flow continuously from posture to posture.

The arrows on the pictures indicate the direction of movement from the previous position into the current one. Study the positions of the arms, legs and body, in relation to both the previous picture and the surroundings, and relate this to the directional arrows and the text describing the movement. Imagine the movements between the images shown, moving from the last posture to the next, along the direction of the arrows.

MOVING THROUGH THE FORM

Apply the principles that you have already learned regarding body alignments, weight shifting, turning, and kwa squat and tuck. Try to coordinate the movements of your arms, legs and body, as you did in the Cloud Hands chi gung exercise. Throughout your t'ai chi form, have a sense of your spine moving as a unit, and being the core of the movement.

Start with at least a short standing practice, allowing your chi to drop into the ground beneath your feet before you begin moving. Once you start moving, proceed at whatever pace you find easiest while maintaining awareness and being physically comfortable with the movements. T'ai chi is generally practised at a slow pace (extremely slow when practised for meditation), but you will want to adopt a medium pace to start with, just slow enough to coordinate your movements. You should expect to take about 5 minutes to complete the short form, once you have learned the movements. Then you can start to slow down, until the form takes about 10 minutes to complete. Once you feel comfortable with this slower pace, you can move as slowly as you wish, while maintaining maximum awareness and not "spacing out". Be aware that the slower you move, the more stamina it will require: faster is generally easier.

KEY PRINCIPLES
The following are some key points to remember:
- Flow continuously through the movements.
- Move your body and limbs as a unit, with the spine directing all movement.
- Direct a relaxed gaze in the direction of your movement.
- Do not cross the centreline of your body with your hands.
- Maintain a sense of heavy elbows and relaxed shoulders.
- Your elbow tips should remain at 45 degrees to the vertical, or lower, pointing at the floor, unless specified.
- Keep your head suspended and your upper body light, while your lower body is relaxed and heavy.
- Keep the space at the base of your skull open, never tipping your head back, especially when leaning forward.
- Never lock any of your joints, either open or closed.
- Keep your weighted knee fixed above the centre of your foot as you turn; do not let your knee joint twist.
- Keep your chest and belly relaxed, but do not slump.
- Keep your head suspended and your spine rising while the front of your body drops.
- Use only as much strength in your arms as you need to hold them in position.
- Keep your hands very relaxed, even when making a fist.
- Do not hold your breath, or impose a breathing pattern. Breathe through your nose, with your tongue gently touching your palate.
- Keep the heel of your back foot on the floor when tucking after a squat.
- When tucking, and at other times, do not force your pelvis and tailbone downwards or forwards.
- Remember to keep within the comfort zone.
- Keep space in your armpits at all times.
- Keep your hands at least a fist-distance from any part of your body, unless otherwise specified.
- Do not try to force your body open. Create space by relaxing, then move into that space.
- Direct your chi to your five points: the top of your head, both palms and the soles of the feet.

Commencement

The following exercise, as well as being the start of the t'ai chi form, is an excellent chi gung practice in its own right. It consists of four sequential movements that can be practised in a continuous cycle. Each of them embodies one of the four main energies of t'ai chi. These are known as "peng" (ward off), "ji" (press), "lu" (roll back) and "an" (push downwards). You can perform "commencement" repeatedly before the main form.

"Peng" energy has a quality like wood floating or a balloon expanding. "Ji" energy is like a spear moving out in a straight line. "Lu" energy is soft and yielding, or like a strong vacuum, and is the characteristic, yin, energy of t'ai chi. "An" energy is heavy and crushing, like a weight dropping. These four energies are different ways of manifesting your central or true chi. The movements of "commencement" enable you to manifest them relatively easily: in the rest of the t'ai chi form, they are applied in more complex ways that are not necessarily as clear-cut. There are four additional energies: "tsai" (pull down), "lieh" (split), "kao" (shoulder stroke) and "jou" (elbow stroke). Tsai is a combination of "lu" and "an", and "lieh" is the combination of "peng" and "ji" energy. The shoulder and elbow strokes bring energy to those parts of the body.

Allow your arms, legs and body to move simultaneously. This principle is described in the t'ai chi classics as: "One part moves, all parts move. One part stops, all parts stop." No part of your body should move in isolation, but you should feel that your whole body moves as one unit. This unifies the chi of your entire body into an integrated whole, and is a very important concept in t'ai chi.

During "commencement", in order of the movements you will be: raising chi from the ground "peng", then extending it into space in front of you "ji", then drawing it back into you "lu", and finally dropping it back into the ground "an".

By alternately bending and opening your limbs and kwa you are forming a cycle from yin to yang and back again. You are also alternately gathering energy and releasing it – again in a yin/yang cycle.

As you begin, you may find it useful to perform this several times before you move into the rest of the form. The function of "commencement" is to "start your engine", getting your chi to start flowing and settling you mentally and physically into your practice. Repeat it as many times as you need, until you feel relaxed and your awareness is connected with your movements and your chi, and then proceed with the rest of the form.

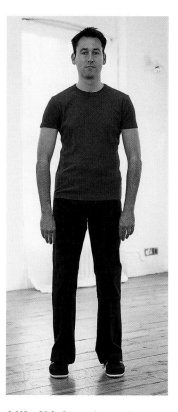

1 Wu Chi Start from the wu chi standing posture. Ideally do at least 10 minutes of standing practice before proceeding. In any case, establish correct t'ai chi alignments, then allow your chi to drop into your tantien, and from there into the ground beneath your feet.

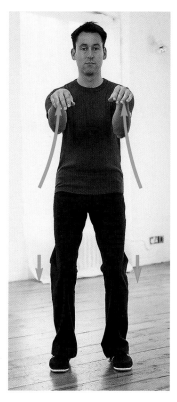

2 Peng Sit into your kwa, allowing your knees to bend as you bring your wrists upwards and outwards in an arc. As your arms rise, keep your wrists totally relaxed and bend your elbow joint, bringing your elbow tips to vertical (pointing at the floor). Your wrists should move in from your sides until they are aligned on your side channels.

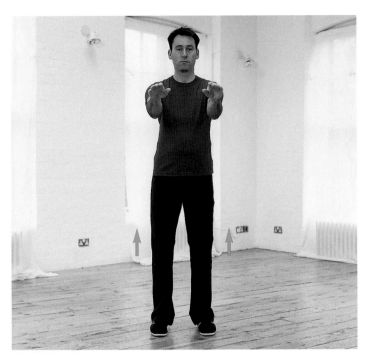

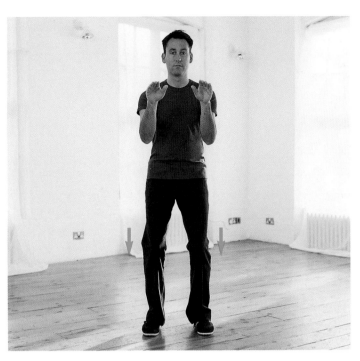

3 Ji Open your kwa and stand up as you unfold your arms in a wave-like motion towards your fingertips. Allow your hands and fingers to open, and keep a 30 per cent bend in your arms and legs. Keep your elbow tips pointing vertically downwards, and your palms facing the ground. Do not raise your chest; soften and hollow your shoulders' nests. Keep your eyes open and gaze in a relaxed way into the space beyond your fingertips.

4 Lu Sit again into your kwa, bending your knees while dropping your elbows vertically, bringing your hands in towards your body at shoulder's nest height. Bring your wrists straight in, to about a fist's distance from your body, keeping your wrist joints completely relaxed. Feel as if you are drawing energy inwards through your fingers. Have a very "empty", yin, mental attitude as you do this: a sense of effortlessly drawing everything into yourself.

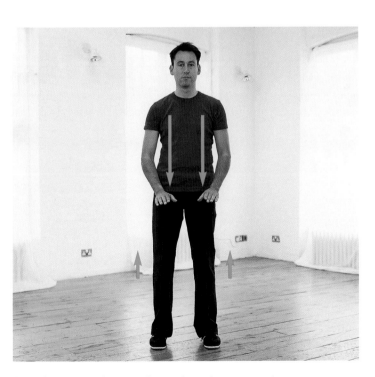

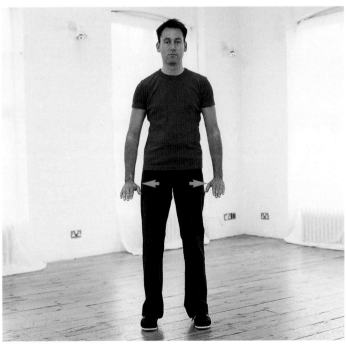

5 An Open your kwa and stand again, as you drop your hands straight down the line of your side channels to the level of your lower tantien, where they move round to your sides; keep your fingers pointing forward and your hands about a fist's distance from your body as you move your chi to the soles of your feet.

6 An Beware of raising your chest during this move. As you stand up, relax and drop your chest. Once you have brought your hands to your sides (by the sides of your legs), then maintain the feeling of dropping your chi for a few moments, then completely relax your hands, going "neutral" and fully releasing your chi beneath your feet.

Raise Hands

With this sequence you begin moving into the main part of the form. You will now start to move your body in more complex patterns. Review the t'ai chi principles set out earlier, and try to incorporate these in all your movements.

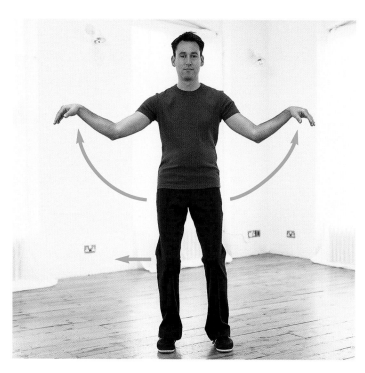

1 Shift your weight to your right, doing "peng" to the sides, wrists rising as your arms and legs bend. Do not pull your arms too far back – your chest should stay relaxed.

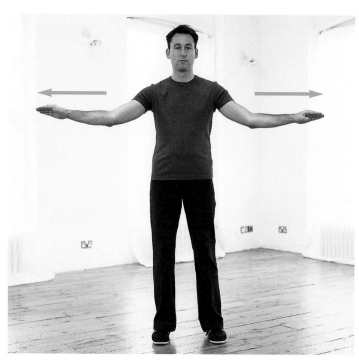

2 Open into "ji" as you stand up, keeping your weight 100 per cent on your right leg. Do not lock your elbows or knees.

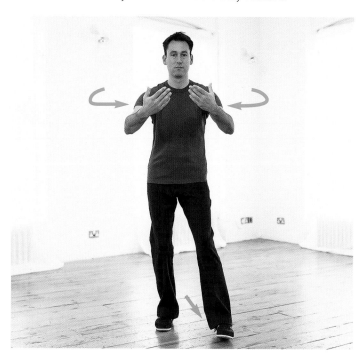

3 Sit into your kwa as you allow your left leg to swing forward, placing your left heel slightly in front of you, toes up. Keep 100 per cent of your weight on your rear leg. Simultaneously bring your arms in front of you in a hugging motion until your palms are aligned with your shoulders' nests. Elbows point downward at 45 degrees: feel as if they are resting on your hips.

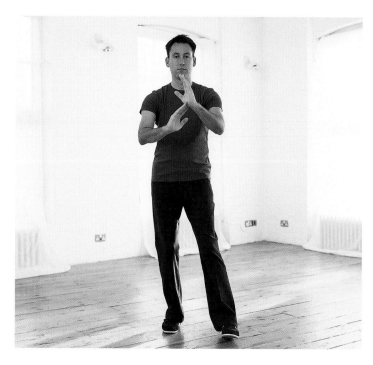

4 Keeping the roundness in your arms, press your palms toward each other on your centreline until you are touching your left pulse with your right fingers. This action opens the space between your shoulder blades. This opening may extend further down your back. As you end the movement, allow the front of your body to relax and sink as your spine rises.

Play the Lute

Here you will start turning your body in coordination with arm and leg movements.
Remember to make all turning originate in the spine, with your arms and legs
turning like the spokes on a wheel (the spine is the axle).

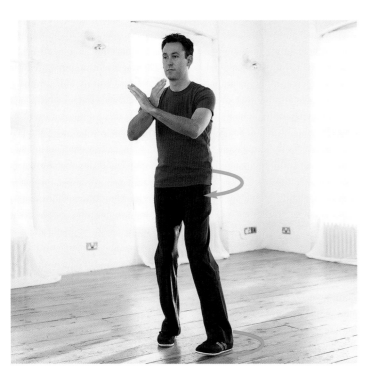

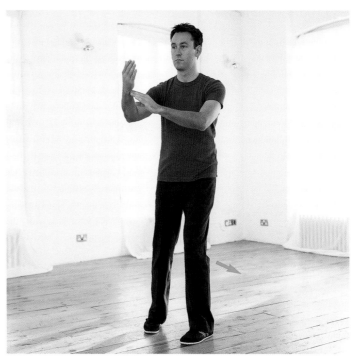

1 Staying rear-weighted, fold into your right kwa as you turn 45 degrees to the right. Allow your left leg to turn with your spine. Slide your left hand underneath your right hand as you turn, so your wrists are crossed.

2 Shift your weight to your left side and slide your right hand over your left hand until you are touching your right pulse with your left fingers. Turn the back of your right hand to face outwards as you move. Look in the direction of your right hand.

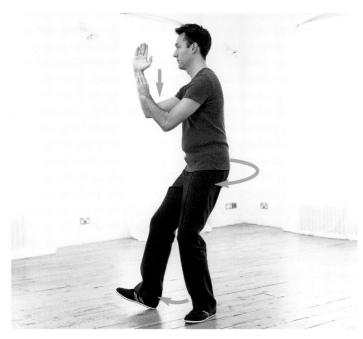

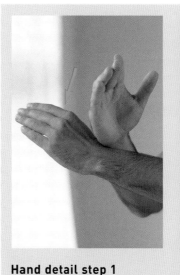

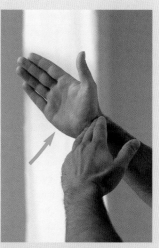

3 Stay left-weighted as you sit into your kwa and turn a further 45 degrees to the right as you allow your right leg to swing in front of you, placing your right heel on the floor slightly in front of you, toes up. Simultaneously drop your elbows as you bring your hands towards you until your right fingers are pointing vertically upwards, at face height and on your centreline.

Hand detail step 1
As you turn your body 45 degrees to the right keep your right hand fixed and slide your left hand underneath it until your wrists are crossed.
Note: this image is a left side view.

Hand detail step 2
As you shift your weight to your left leg (body still turned 45 degrees to the right) keep your left hand fixed and slide your right hand over your left.
Note: this image shows your point of view.

Grasp Sparrow's Tail

This sequence incorporates all the main energies of t'ai chi. In sequence, you will do "peng", "lu", "ji", "lu" and "an" energy. This will give you a feeling for the way in which you transform your chi as you move through the form.

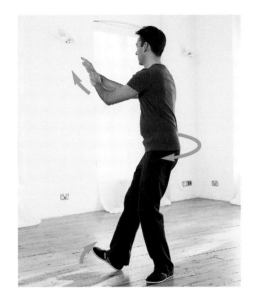

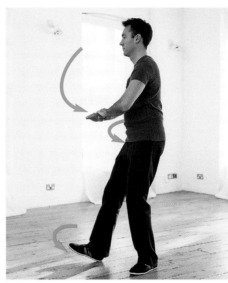

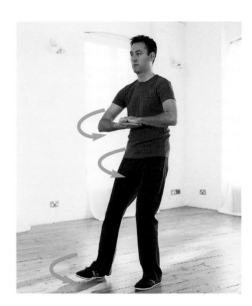

1 Staying rear-weighted (left leg), open your kwa and limbs as you turn 45 degrees to the right, touching the back of your right wrist with your left fingers as your hands move out and up in a clockwise circle. Turn your right leg with your body. Feel that you are expanding your energy outwards ("peng" energy).

2 Turn back to the left (staying rear-weighted) as you bring your hands in and down towards you, sliding your right hand under your left. Feel that you are drawing energy inwards ("lu" energy).

3 Continue turning to the left until you are almost fully folded into your left kwa. Your forearms should finish in a straight line, with the right palm over the back of the left hand. Your hands should be no lower than your elbows in order to release your shoulders and neck.

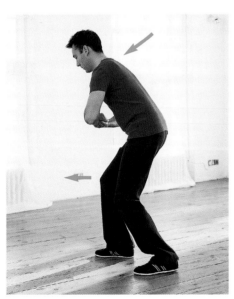

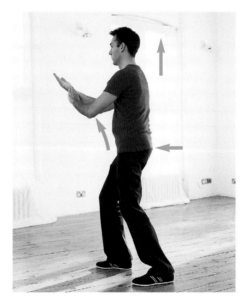

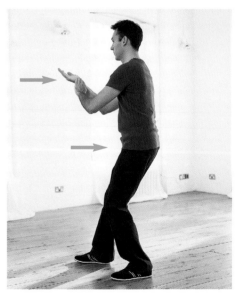

4 Turn your right palm upwards and turn your centre 45 degrees to the right (90 degrees from the commencement position). Shift 100 per cent of your weight to your front (right) leg and squat into your kwa, keeping your palms together. Reposition your back foot so that your stance is comfortable.

5 Stand up on your front leg – without shifting your weight back – as you open your kwa and tuck your pelvis. Touching your right pulse, "scissor" your arms up and out to heart height with the centres of your palms on your centreline. Release your energy in a straight line into space in front of you ("ji" energy).

6 Shift your weight to your back leg, sitting into your kwa as you allow your elbows to drop and fold, still touching your right pulse. Allow your right wrist to relax completely as you move back, as if carrying a plate on your palm. Feel that you are drawing energy inwards ("lu" energy) through your hands.

Alternative View steps 4, 5 and 6

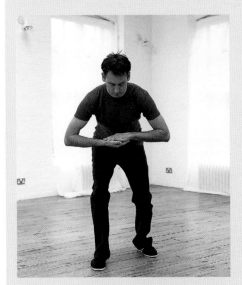 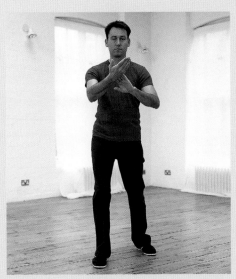 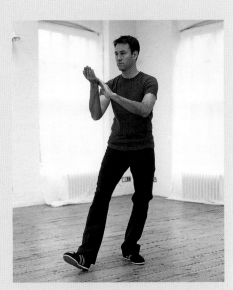

4 Squatting as you gather energy. Note that the hands remain on the centreline of the body. The head is not tipped back, but looking downwards.

5 The posture "ji". Note the centre of the hands are on the centreline of the body at heart height, the arms at 45 degree angles, hands also inclined.

6 Drawing chi in with "lu". Note the 45 degree outward turn, dropped elbows and relaxed wrists. The hands are still on the centreline of the body.

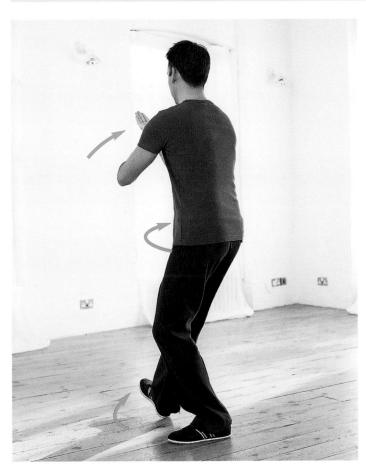 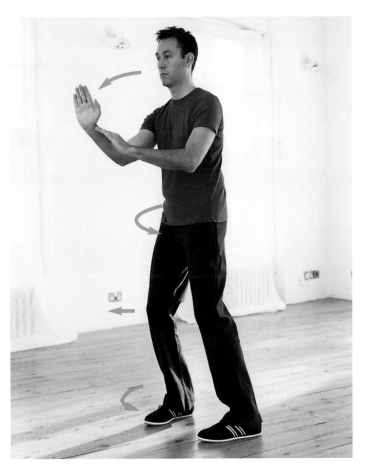

7 Once fully back-weighted (left leg), turn your centre 45 degrees to the right, keeping your hands on your centreline. Maintain the feeling of turning from your spine, with your unweighted leg and your arms linked, like the spokes on a wheel (the spine is the centre of the wheel).

8 Flip your right palm vertically and turn a total of 90 degrees to the left, turning your right foot with your body. Keep your hands on your centreline as you turn. When you are fully turned, shift weight to your right leg as you push heavily ("an" energy) from the heel of your palm and forearm. Do not overextend your arms.

Single Whip

Along with "fan through the back", this is the most open posture in the form, and it allows for the release of not only physical tightness and contraction, but also energetic tension. It is a meditation point, so take a few moments to relax fully once you are in the final posture.

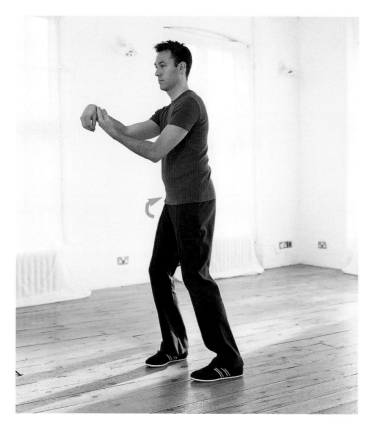

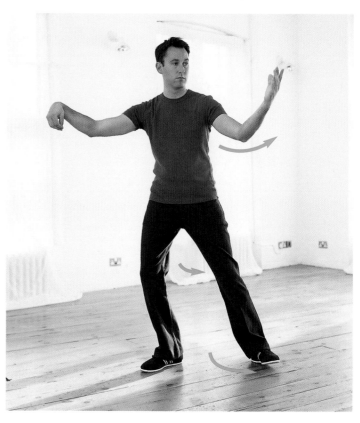

1 Form a "beak" with your right hand by bringing the fingertips together as shown in the hand detail box below, turning your left palm to face you and touching your right pulse. As you do this, "wind up" slightly into your right leg (turning very slightly to the right), with no weight on the left.

2 Releasing the "wind-up", open your body from your centre. Your right hand and right knee should not move at all. Your left hand and left foot move outwards in an arc together. Allow your back to open out and your elbows to move slightly away from your spine.

Hand Detail step 1

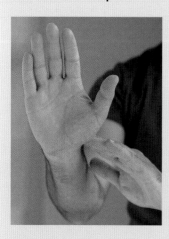

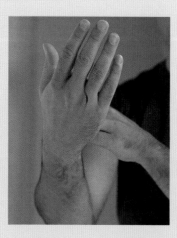

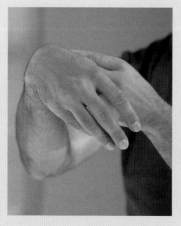

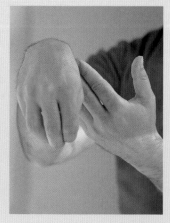

The final hand position of the previous posture (double "an" within "grasp sparrow's tail")

Turn the palms of both hands towards you.

Circle your right hand anticlockwise, leading with the little finger.

Finish with your right hand dropped, wrist relaxed, and all four fingers touching the thumb, forming a beak.

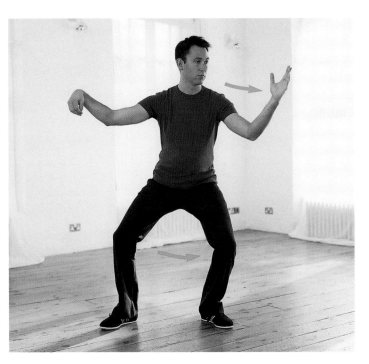

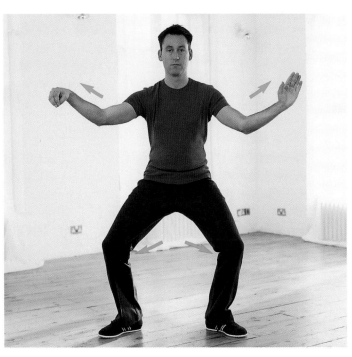

3 Shift your weight to the left, as you fold slightly into your left kwa. The edge of your left hand points in the same direction as your left foot.

4 Shift and turn to the centre (evenly weighted left/right). Keep your hands at or below shoulder height, elbows dropped. Sit into your legs, keeping your spine straight. Release outwards.

Diagonal Flying and Hold Ball

"Diagonal flying" moves chi from one extremity of your body to the other, lengthening the body. "Hold ball" develops the ability to issue chi from your hands.

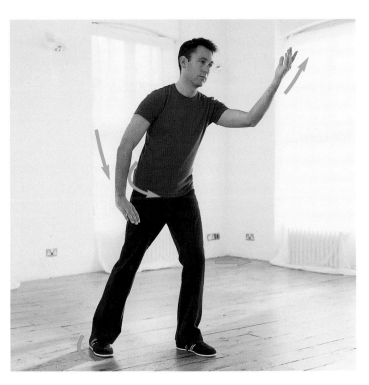

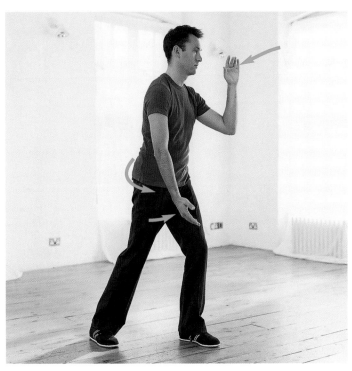

1 Shift your weight to the left. Turn 45 degrees to the left, swivelling your right foot on the heel to point in the same direction as your left foot. Simultaneously turn your left hand palm up, and bring your right hand palm down to the level of your right kwa. Feel as if you are pushing energy down with the right hand, which then rises up and out of your left arm.

2 Staying left-weighted, wind up a little into your left leg (into your left kwa) as you turn your hands over, left palm down, right palm up, as if holding a large ball. Allow your right hand to move slightly left to your centreline. Feel as if your palms are energetically connected to one another.

Yin Release and Shoulder Stroke

The "yin release" posture releases and drains the yin channels of the front of the body, and is highly effective when used as a standing posture for stress relief. "Shoulder stroke" opens the pelvis, and is one of the main martial moves of t'ai chi.

As the front of your body "sinks" in the first move of this sequence, allow your spine to rise proportionally. This activates the "microcosmic orbit" of energy within you, which is a naturally occurring circuit of chi that goes down the front of the body, loops through the tantien and perineum, and up the spine and over the head. The descending phase of this circuit is yin, and the ascending is yang. The place where your tongue touches the palate (roof of the mouth) is the changeover point, and acts as a switch to allow the chi to flow more strongly. It is for this reason that you should have your tongue touching your palate the entire time you are practising t'ai chi or chi gung.

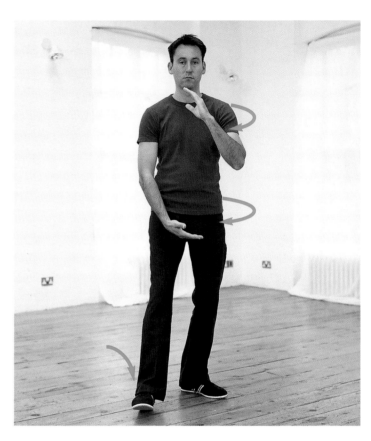

1 Keeping your right hand fixed in position, and your weight on your left leg, turn your centre 45 degrees to the right and allow the right leg to swing in front of you, placing your right heel on the floor slightly in front of you, toes up. Relax the inside of your right arm and your chest as you turn. Bring your left hand around with your centre, to finish with it in front of your heart (or throat), directly above your lower (right) hand, which is in front of your tantien. Relax the entire front of your body, from the crown of your head down to your toes, allowing all tension and blockage to melt downwards into the ground.

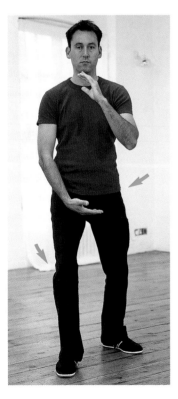

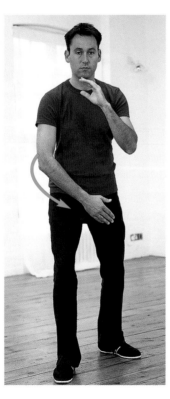

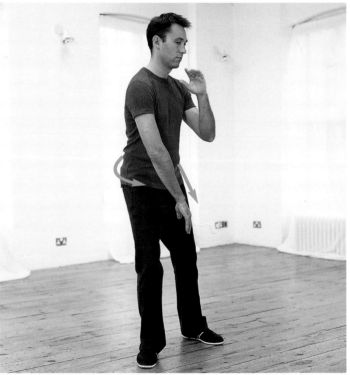

2 Shift your weight to your front (right) foot. Then open your right kwa as you turn your centre 45 degrees to the left, spiralling your right hand downwards to open your right shoulder blade.

3 Keep your right knee fixed, kneecap facing forwards as you turn. Your right hip and right shoulder should move forward (in the direction of your knee) as you turn. Keep your head suspended and spine upright.

Elbow Strike and Wrist Strike

Another main martial technique, "elbow strike" follows "shoulder stroke" in a wavelike motion, finishing at the end of the arm with "wrist strike". These postures will help move chi from your spine through your arm to your fingertips.

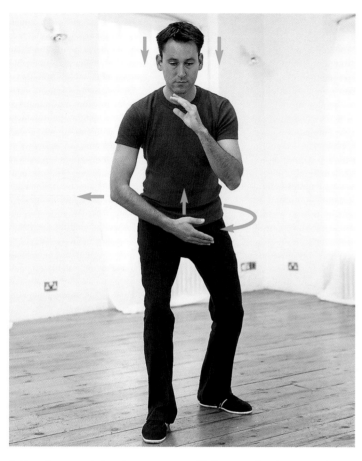

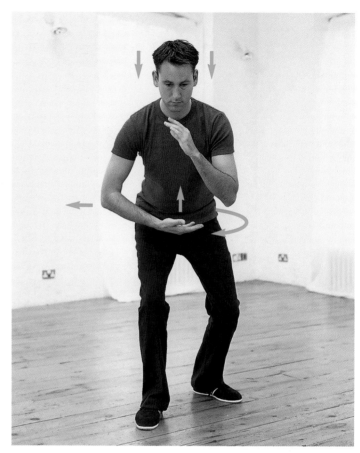

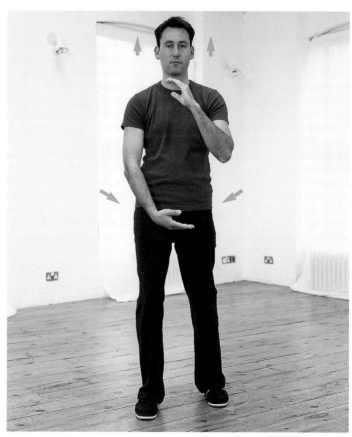

1 Stay front-weighted as you turn 45 degrees back to the right and squat into your kwa, while bringing your right hand up your centreline, turning your palm upwards as you move. Bring your left hand with your centreline as you turn.

2 As you turn and squat your right hand proportionally spirals up your centreline. This will bring your elbow out to your right side and energize it. When you have completed the move, while squatting, reposition your back leg closer to you with your back foot parallel to your front foot.

3 Stand up while remaining fully weighted on your right leg (tucking your pelvis under you), keeping your back foot on the floor. As you rise, allow your right hand to move out in front of your tantien, as if tossing a coin away. Keep your left hand on your centreline. If you cannot keep your back foot on the floor, this means your stance is too long and you should bring your rear foot further forward. This a general rule in t'ai chi. Over time, your leg sinews will lengthen and release and you will be able to adopt a longer stance.

White Crane Spreads Its Wings

This posture moves chi both up and down your centreline simultaneously. Overall the shape your hands make is like a smooth rectangle: up your centre, across the top to the right, down the right, across the bottom, up the left and back to the centre.

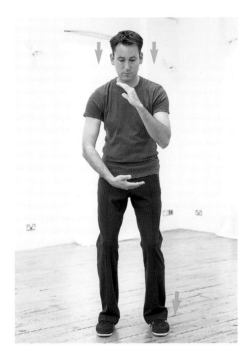

1 Sit in your kwa, drawing up your rear foot to bring it parallel to your front foot, normal standing width apart.

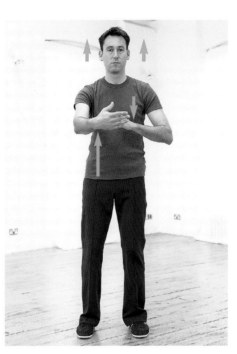

2 Return to an upright position, while dropping your left hand down your centreline and bringing your right hand up your centreline, in front of your left hand. Continue moving your arms as you drop your weight down your left side.

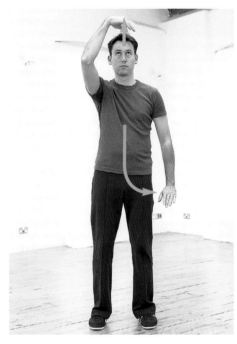

3 When your left hand reaches your lower tantien it should move round to your left side. Your right hand finishes above your head. Look upwards at your right hand as it rises (without tipping your head back). Weight is on the left leg.

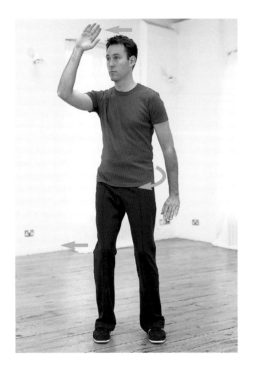

4 Shift your weight to the right and turn into your right kwa. Keep your left hand fixed by your left side, and bring your right hand to your centre as you turn.

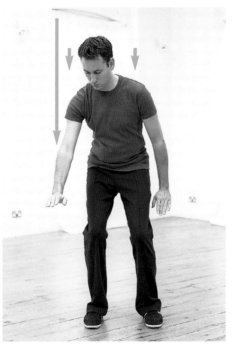

5 Still turned to the right, squat into your kwa evenly on both sides and lower your right arm until it is at thigh height, fingers pointing forward.

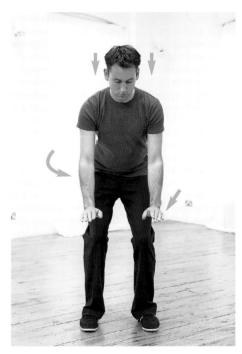

6 Turn and shift your weight back to the centre as you slide your left hand forward, to finish parallel with your right hand and at the same height.

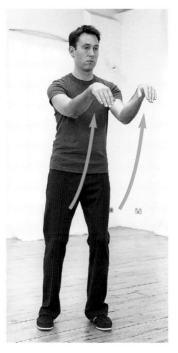

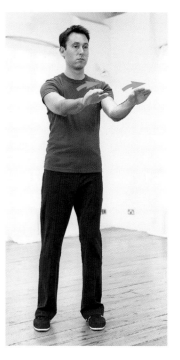

8 Remaining turned to the left, stand as you do "peng".

9 Open into "ji", still turned to the left.

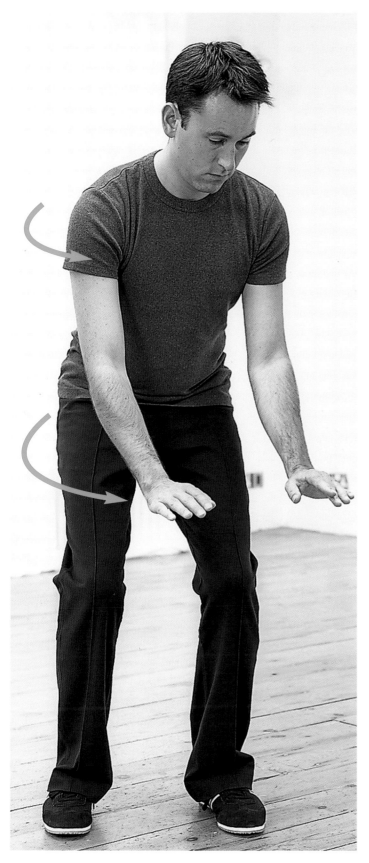

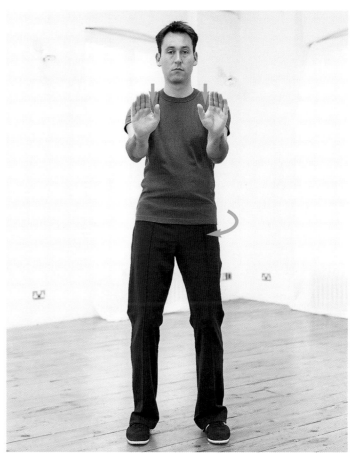

7 Shift your weight to the left and turn into your left kwa, keeping your arms linked to your spine. You knees should not twist at all, keeping the space between your legs. You may find you can make only a very small turn here.

10 Turn back to the centre as you "sit in the wrists", drawing energy in through your fingertips, down your arms (allowing your elbows to sink), into your spine and down through your body. As you sit in the wrists, allow your pelvis to relax and drop, while keeping your head suspended. This increases the space between your spinal vertebrae.

Brush Knee and Twist Step

In this sequence you will perform the same movements alternately on your right and left sides, a total of three times. It is excellent for opening your shoulders and hips and developing good balance and left/right coordination.

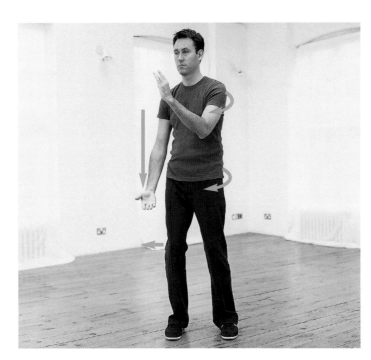

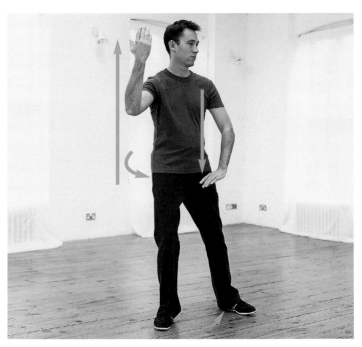

1 Shift your weight to the right and turn 45 degrees into your right kwa, as you bring your right hand down to your right side, palm up, bringing your left hand to your centre, palm facing to the right.

2 With your weight on your right leg, open your right kwa and turn your centre 90 degrees to the left, bringing your left heel in an arc, slightly behind your right heel. At the same time, bring your right hand up to ear height, palm facing you, and your left hand down your centreline, palm down at tantien height. Your left foot points in the same direction as your centre.

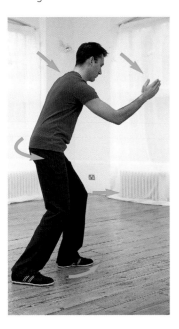 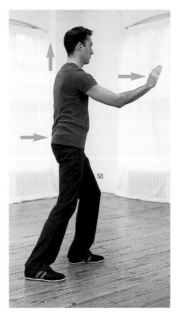

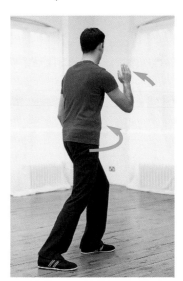 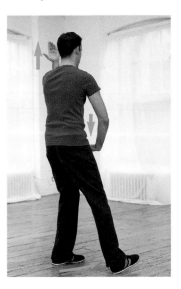

3 Turn your centre and your left foot (swivelling on the heel) a further 45 degrees to the left, bringing your left hand to the side of your left leg. Transfer your weight to your left leg and squat into your left kwa, bringing your right arm down and forwards in front of you, fingers pointing forwards. Reposition your right foot closer and parallel to your left foot. Stand up on your left leg (tucking your pelvis), turning your right hand palm out as if pushing forwards, keeping your elbow tip down.

4 Keep your weight on your left leg and turn 45 degrees into your left kwa, bringing your right hand across to your centre, palm facing left, and turning your left hand over, palm up, as if holding a large ball at your side. Stay turned to the left and step through with your right foot, resting your right heel on the floor in front of you, foot angled with your turn. Stand up, your left hand rising to ear height, palm facing you, your right hand moving down your centreline, palm down at tantien height.

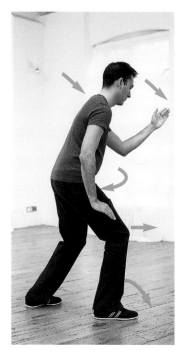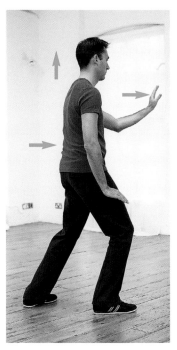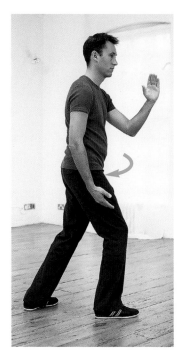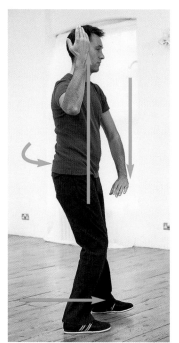

5 Staying rear-weighted, turn your centre and your right foot (swivelling on the heel) 45 degrees to the right, bringing your right hand to the side of your leg. Transfer your weight to your right leg and squat into your kwa as you bring your left arm down and forwards in front of you, fingers pointing forwards.

6 Stand up on your right leg, and turn your left hand palm out, keeping your elbow tip pointing vertically down.

7 Keep your weight on your right leg and turn 45 degrees into your right kwa, bringing your left hand across to your centreline, palm facing right, and turning your right hand over, palm up, as if holding a large ball at your side.

8, 9, 10 Continue the sequence from here in a mirror image of what you did on the left side, until you finish with your left foot forward, pushing with your right palm.

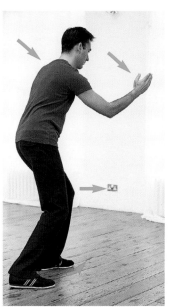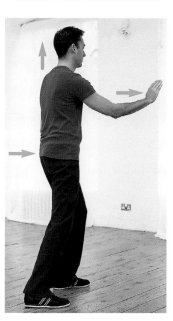

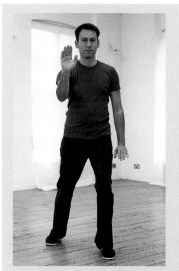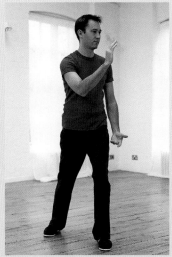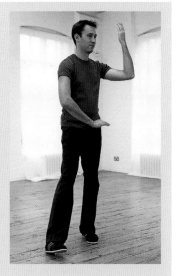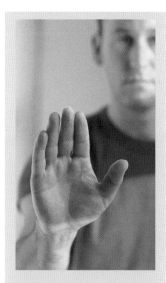

Alternative View steps 3 and 4
Tucking and pushing forward, turning to the left and holding a ball, stepping through.

Hand detail step 3
A relaxed and open hand.

Needle at Sea Bottom

In this sequence, you will first send your energy straight upwards, above your head, and then straight downwards into the ground. This move will help strengthen your legs and release your kwa, hips and sacrum.

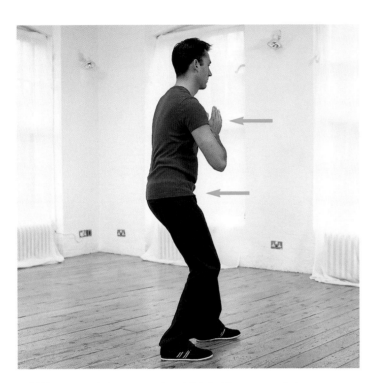

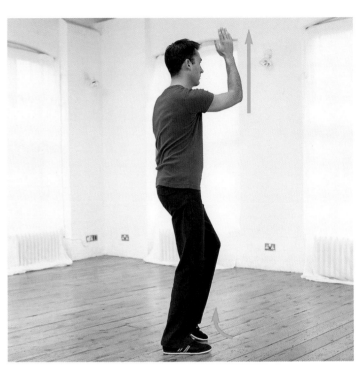

1 Shift your weight to your back (right) leg as you bring your right hand in towards your heart (palm facing left), keeping your left hand, palm down, by your side, and sit into your kwa.

2 With a sense of pushing energy down with the left hand and pushing downwards with your tailbone through your right (weighted) heel, open your kwa and limbs as your body rises and your right hand ascends your centreline to finish above (and in front of) your head. At the same time, lift your unweighted left heel until only your left toes touch the ground. Follow the right hand with your eyes; do not tip your head back.

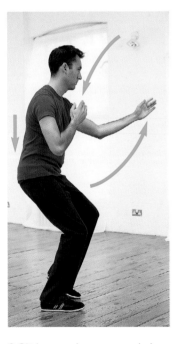

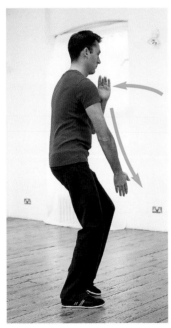

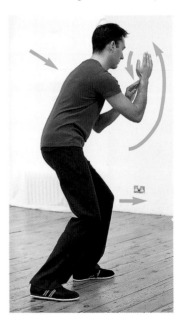

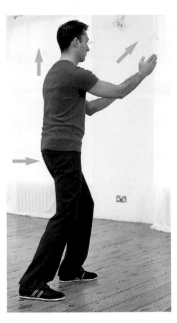

3 Sit in your kwa as you bring your right hand downwards and your left hand out and up, as if your hands are circling each other, palms facing. At the point where you are fully sitting in your kwa, your hands are at the same height. Open your kwa, but not your legs, as your right hand continues downwards on your centreline, fingers pointing down and your left hand rounds the top of the circle and moves in towards your heart.

4 Shift the weight to your left foot and squat as your hands circle to bring your left fingers to your right pulse. Your arms and legs bend at the same time. Tuck your pelvis and stand up on your left leg, stabbing your right fingers upwards.

Alternative View Needle at Sea Bottom

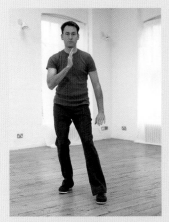

1 The left hand remains by your side as you move.

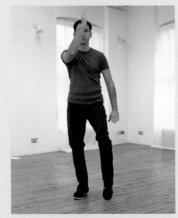

2 Your right hand ascends your centreline.

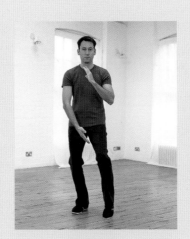

3 Opening the kwa as the right hand descends.

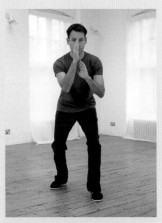

4 Squatting on the front leg as your hands join.

Fan Through the Back

Along with "single whip", "fan through the back" is the most open posture in the form, and is a meditation point where you allow complete release of your body and mind.

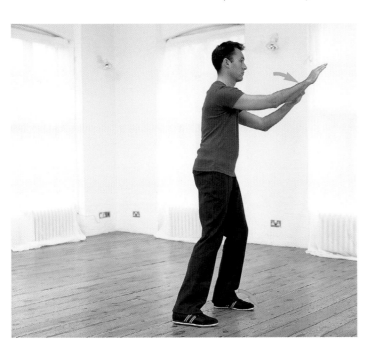

1 Without shifting your weight, turn your left foot and centre 45 degrees to the right. Stay weighted on your left leg. Bring your arms with your turn, and turn your right hand palm down.

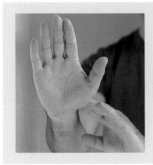

Hand Detail step 1

Gently touching the back of your right wrist with your left hand. As you open in step 2, your left hand will remain fixed and your right hand will move with your body until you finish in the position shown in 2.

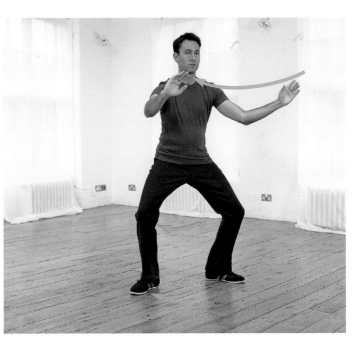

2 Keeping your left hand fixed in space above your left leg, open your body from the centre, bringing your lower body into an identical position to "single whip" (centre-weighted), but with your arms asymmetrical: your left hand in line with your left knee and your right hand aligned with your right shoulder's nest. Both hands should be at the same height and the same distance from your body. Feel as if you are drawing a bow as you move: your left hand is holding the bow (fixed), and your right hand is drawing the bowstring. As you finish in the central position, allow your arms to release outwards from your spine, opening your body from the centre, as if letting the arrow fly. Eventually you should also feel that your legs release in the same way. Release your central channel as in "single whip".

Turn and Chop with Back of Fist

This sequence will give you a strong sense of alternately opening your body, closing it, and opening it again. It will help you be aware of your centre, and develop stability and balance while turning.

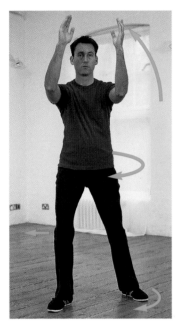 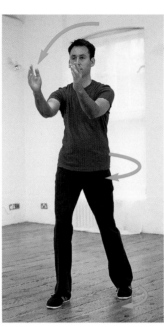 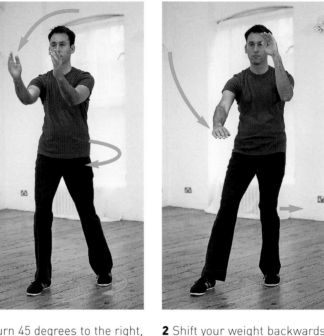 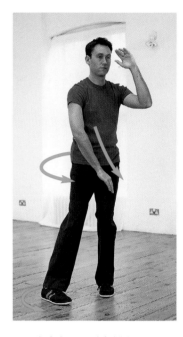

1 Shift your weight to the right and turn 45 degrees to the right, swivelling your unweighted left foot on the heel to point in the same direction as your right foot. Simultaneously move both your hands up, inwards and down in an arc until your arms are parallel in front of you, elbows down and palms facing each other at shoulder height, at the width of your side channels.

2 Shift your weight backwards to your left leg and fold into your left kwa, swivelling your right foot on the heel. Feel as if you are folding into your centre. Allow your left hand to follow your centreline as you move, and your right arm to spiral down to finish with your hand in front of your tantien. This is the most closed posture in the form. Your right foot turns inwards.

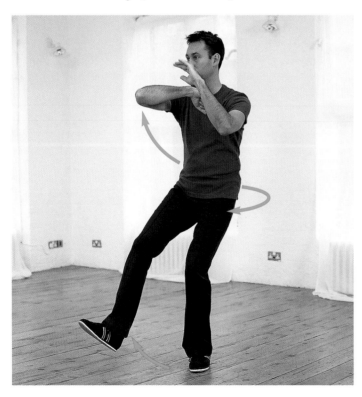 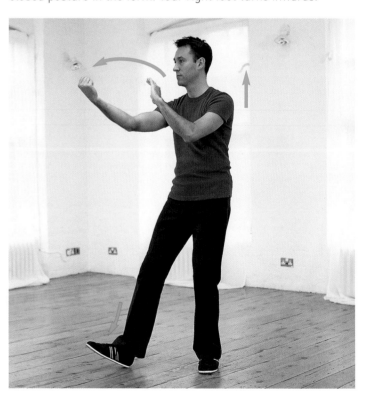

3 Staying weighted on your left leg, open your left kwa, lifting your right foot off the floor, as you turn your centre 90 degrees to the right. As you move, strike outwards with your right elbow.

4 Unfold your arm and strike out with the back of your (relaxed) fist as your right heel touches down. Your left palm projects chi into your right fist.

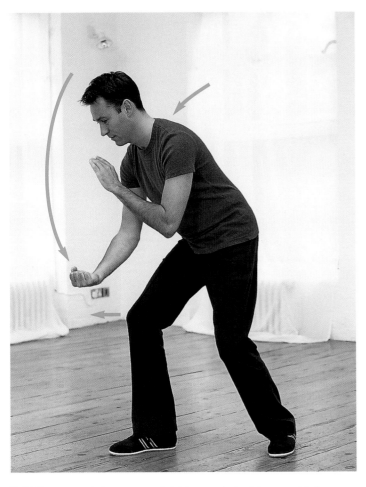

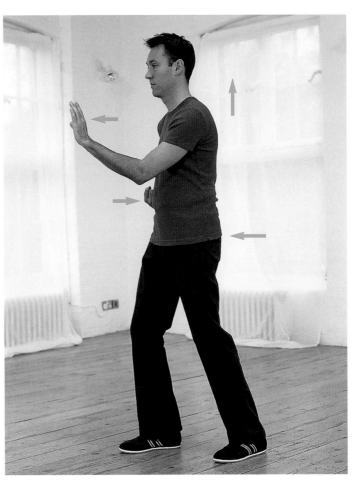

5 Shift your weight to your right leg and start to squat into your kwa. Reposition your back foot when necessary. As you squat, bring your right fist down your centreline, as if it is very heavy ("an" energy).

6 When you are reaching the limit of your squat, start tucking and standing up again, weight on your front leg. Your right fist arcs upwards, to finish at your side just above your hip bone. Your left hand turns outwards in front of your heart, as if you are pushing something away from you.

Alternative View steps 4, 5 and 6

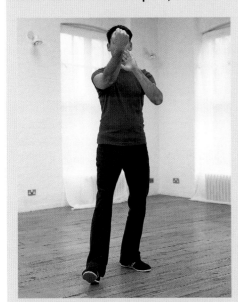

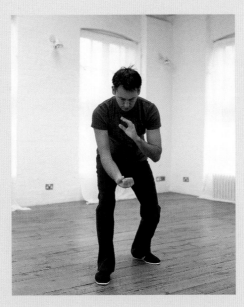

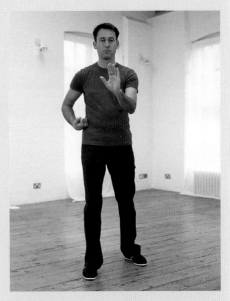

4 As you chop outwards with the back of your fist it remains on your centreline. In martial terms, the front heel is stamping to a shin or instep.

5 Keeping both hands on your centreline as you shift your weight forward and squat. Make sure your head does not tip backwards.

6 Tucking and standing up on your front leg, right fist at the top of the hip/base of the liver, and left hand on the centreline in front of the heart.

Parry and Punch

During the following movements, up to the punch, your right fist continuously circles your liver. This releases energetic blockage in that organ. Keep the contact between the side of your fist and your body very relaxed and light.

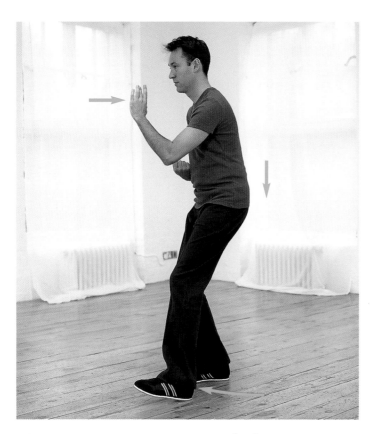

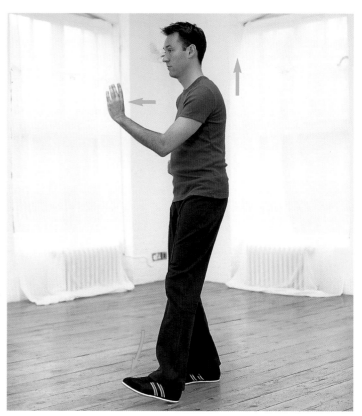

1 Sit into your kwa and swing your back (left) leg forwards until your left heel is resting on the floor in front of you. At the same time, bring your left hand in towards your heart.

2 Stand up on your right leg, opening your kwa, and push out in front of your heart with the outside edge of your left hand, gently pushing downwards with your left heel.

3 Staying on your back leg, lengthen from your left foot, up your left leg, through your body and along your left arm to the tips of your fingers, allowing your left hand to move outwards and your body to turn naturally to the right.

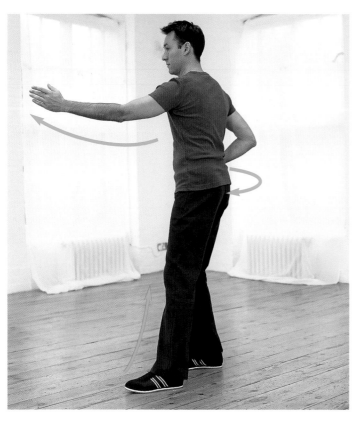

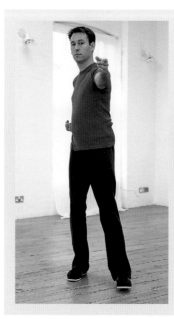

Alternative View step 3
Keep your back leg stable and rooted as you lengthen up from your front (left) leg, through the left side, and along your left arm to your fingertips.
This will naturally cause your spine to rotate to the right. Allow your head to turn with your spine, but gaze in the direction of your left hand.
Do not lock your left elbow - keep a 30 per cent bend.

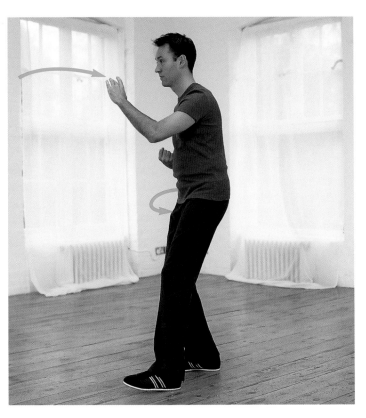

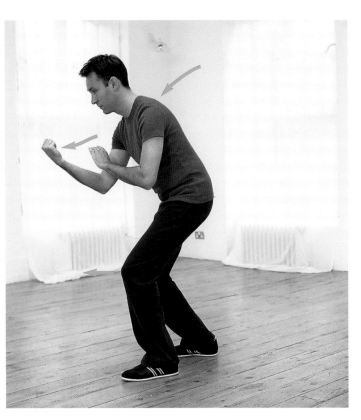

4 Bring your left hand back in towards you and turn your centre back to the left. Your right fist continues to circle your liver as you are moving.

5 Shift your weight to the left leg and squat into that side, repositioning your rear (right) foot when necessary. As you squat, bring your circling right fist downwards and forwards, bending the elbow, fist still turned fingers up.

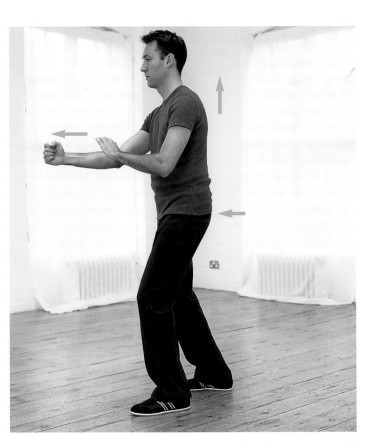

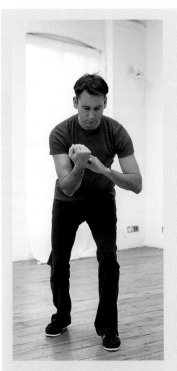

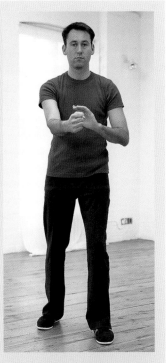

6 Tuck and stand on your left leg as you unbend your arms and legs, allowing your fist to move out and turn over, thumb up, on your centreline. Project chi from your left palm into your right fist. Keep your fist (and your mind) very relaxed at all times.

Alternative View step 5
Shifting to the front leg, preparing for the punch. Your elbow moves downwards and forwards as you squat.

Alternative View step 6
As you tuck and stand up on your front leg, your elbow unbends in proportion to your legs, hips pushing your arm forwards.

Close Up and Step Forward

This sequence involves the closing and opening of your centre, and then the washing downwards of chi through your side channels. This helps clear any stagnation in your chi, first through the horizontal, and then through the vertical line of your body.

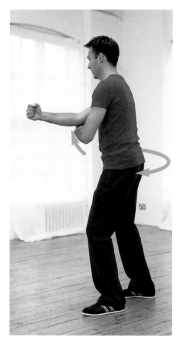

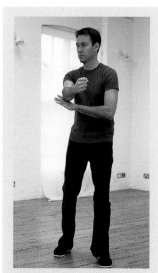

Alternative View
Keep your front (left) knee fixed as you turn.

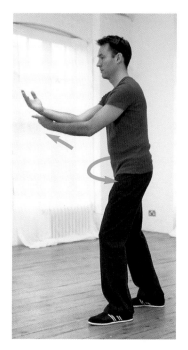

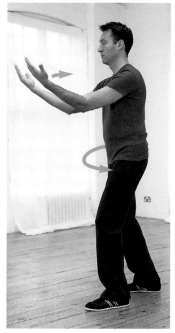

1 Keeping your right fist fixed in space, and your weight on your left leg, open your left kwa and fold into your right kwa, turning your centre to the right without moving your right fist at all. This requires you to relax the inside of your right arm and your chest as you turn. Bring your left hand with your turn, on your centreline, until your left fingers are partly under your right arm, behind the elbow.

2 Open up again, turning back to the left, as you wipe along the underside of your right arm with your left hand, turning both left and right palms upwards as you turn. Finish with palms up at shoulder height, elbows down, on your side channels.

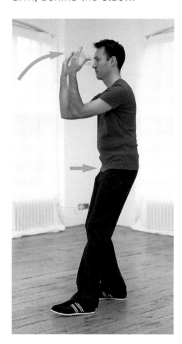

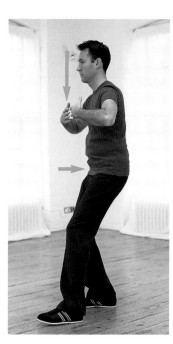

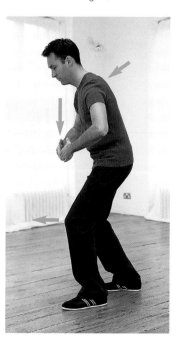

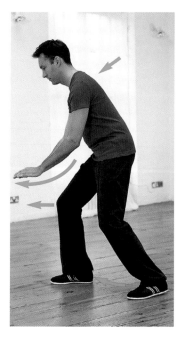

3 Shift your weight back, sitting into your kwa, bringing your palms towards you, keeping your elbows fixed.

4 Take your elbows out to the sides, turning your hands around your laogung points. Allow your shoulders to open.

5 Shift your weight forwards as you bring your hands down your side channels, as if washing downwards through your body. Keep your shoulders relaxed. As you shift forwards fully, step through with your rear (right) leg and shift your weight on to it, squatting as you do so. As you step through, your hands wash down to tantien level, and then turn, fingers forwards, palms down, to release your energy outwards and downwards.

Tiger and Leopard Spring to Mountain

During this sequence, you tuck your pelvis three times in a row, moving it forward progressively more with each tuck. Over time, this will help release tension in your sacrum and tailbone, as long as it is performed gently and without strain.

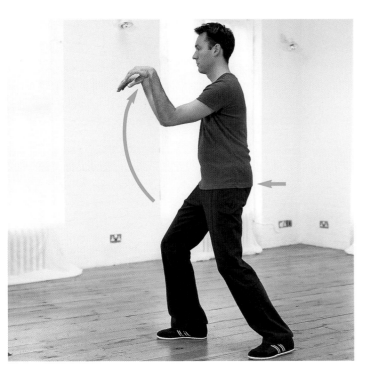

1 Keep your weight on your right leg and tuck slightly, doing "peng" as you did in the "commencement", but keeping 100% of your weight on your front leg.

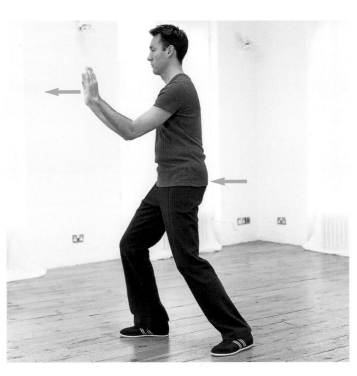

2 Drop into your front leg without bringing your pelvis back, and sit in your wrists, bringing your palms to vertical as if sliding them down a sheet of glass. Tuck again and open your palms, especially the kou area between thumb and index finger. Allow chi to issue from your laogung point, in the centre of your palm.

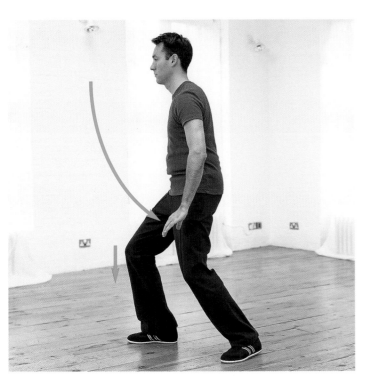

3 Drop again into your front leg (without bringing your pelvis back), and pull your hands downwards and back to your sides, doing "tsai" (pull down).

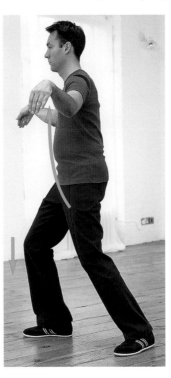

4 As you drop into your front leg, raise your wrists, doing "peng" to the side.

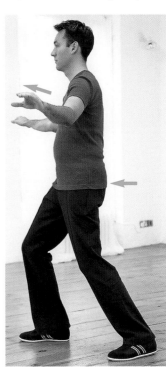

5 Tuck a third time as you do "ji" to the side.

Closing

This is the final part of the form, as you return to the same place on the floor that you started from. As you turn, remember the concept of making your spine the axle of a wheel, with your arms being the spokes that are attached.

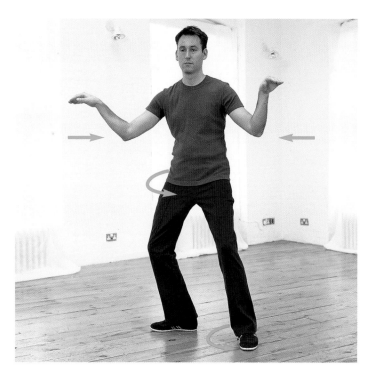

1 Staying weighted on your right leg, open your right kwa and turn your centre 90 degrees to the left (to your starting direction), swivelling on your left heel. As you turn, proportionally pull your hands inwards, dropping your elbows and pulling energy into your spine ("lu").

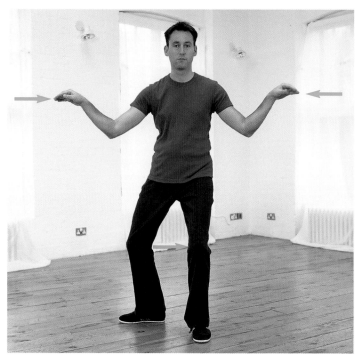

2 When you have turned fully, transfer your weight to your left leg, and start closing into your left kwa as you swivel your unweighted right foot to point in the same direction as your left. Continue to pull in with your arms as you move.

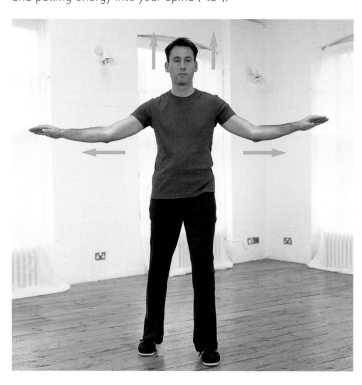

3 Open your kwa and unbend your limbs, doing "ji" to the side.

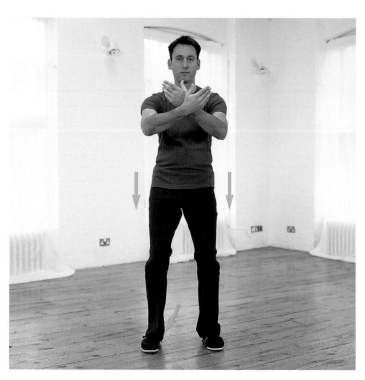

4 Sit into your kwa and slide your rear (right) foot forward, parallel to your left, at shoulder width. As you do this, your arms hug until your wrists are crossed.

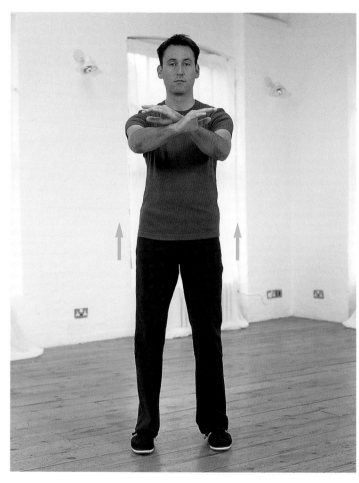

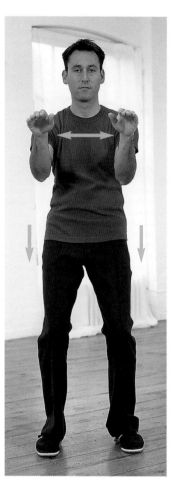

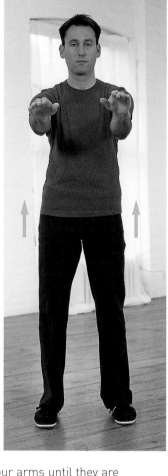

5 Stand up, opening your kwa, moving your weight to the centre and widening the circle of your arms from your spine, keeping your wrists crossed.

6 Sit in your kwa and separate your arms until they are parallel, wrists relaxed. Feel that the outside edges of your hands and forearms are energized with "peng" (horizontal peng). Then do "ji" straight ahead (as in "commencement").

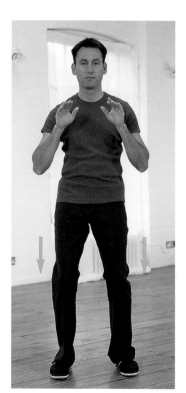

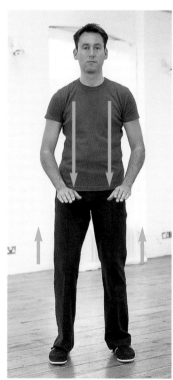

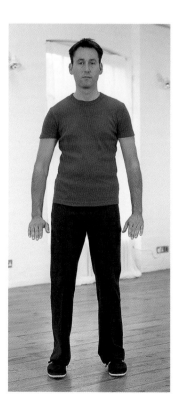

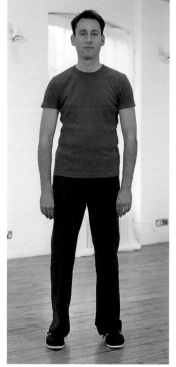

7 Perform "lu" and "an" exactly as in "commencement".

8 Finish your practice in the same wu chi standing posture you began in at the start of the form.

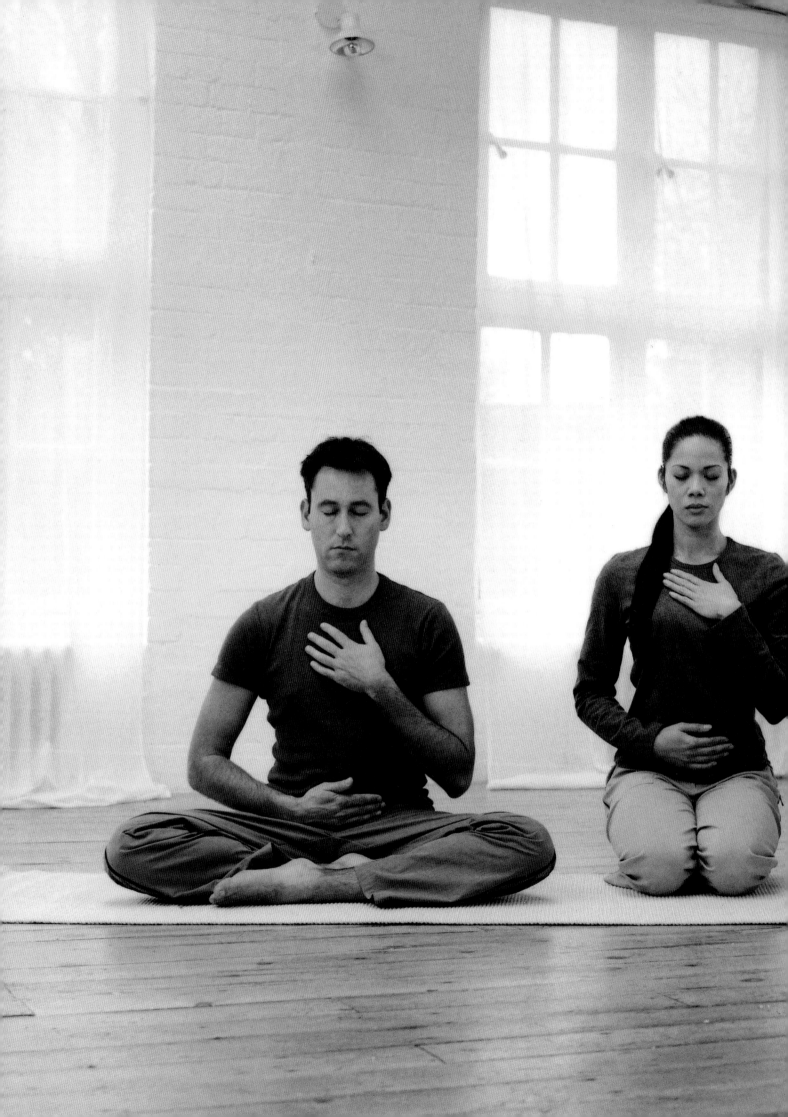

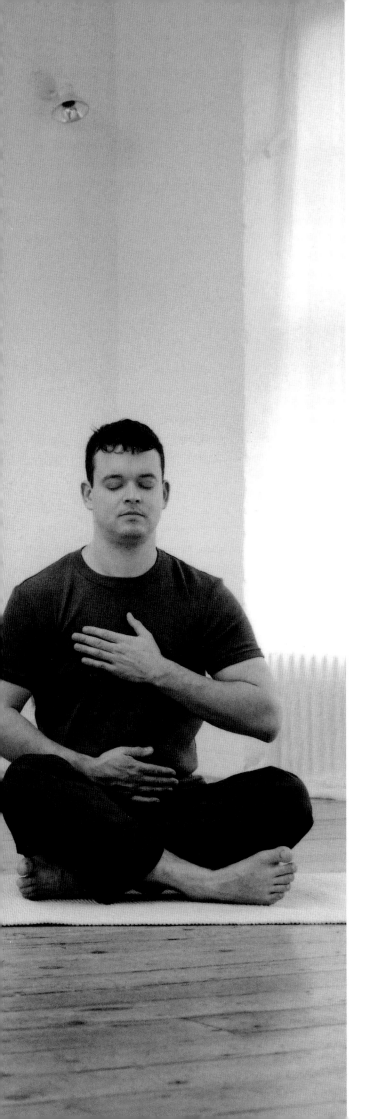

Taking it Further

Your practice can develop and deepen perfectly well using just the short form, because the essence of t'ai chi is to be found in the Taoist nei gung principles, which can be learned and applied fully in the short form. Eventually you may wish to learn a long form, as the repetition and flow can allow for greater development of your chi. However, for a beginner, learning a long form can be a daunting undertaking, and a short form is also far more practical for busy people with little free time. Other practices that take your t'ai chi experience further are push hands and meditation. These will not only help your t'ai chi develop, but are powerful techniques for your personal development. When practised side by side, they can assist you in the process of releasing emotional tensions and even in dealing with ego-related issues. In this respect they can be linked to spiritual practice, and assist on that path.

When and How to Practise

Progress in t'ai chi comes through regular and sustained practice. How much or how little you train depends on how quickly you wish to progress and how much opportunity you have for practice, but some practice is always better than none. Daily practice, even for short sessions, is far more useful than occasional marathons, because it will help integrate t'ai chi principles into your mind, nervous system and body far more easily.

Forging the link between your awareness and your energy is a gradual and sustained process, but very little time is actually needed on a daily basis. If you do have a gap in your regular practice, restart at the last point you felt confident.

EXPERIENCING CHI

At first, you may not feel your chi moving during practice. This is normal. It is often said that it takes six months to a year to "wake up" your chi. This is not an all-or-nothing experience; your awareness of chi develops and deepens over time and there is no end point. Even if you cannot feel chi moving during your practice, it will be; it is taking place below the level of your conscious awareness. If you persevere, you will become consciously aware of your chi, and at that point you can start to work with it more directly. How you experience chi is individual: you may feel sensations such as heat, magnetism, wind, cold, static electricity or tingling, and all are equally valid. The important thing is that you are feeling something. The specific sensations you encounter will vary from day to day, minute to minute, and posture to posture. Try to avoid attaching any great significance to these sensations, and simply be present in the experience.

DEVELOPING YOUR SKILLS

Patience is truly a virtue in learning t'ai chi. Certain t'ai chi skills will take time to develop, no matter how intensively you practise, just as it takes a set time to digest a meal, and this cannot be rushed. As you practise, you will have moments where you gain abilities, or your body or mind release, only to lose that experience again. This "now you see it now you don't" experience is perfectly normal, and over time you will "see it" more than you don't, until that particular ability or experience becomes commonplace to you. Patience and perseverance will always yield results.

Learning t'ai chi is like learning to drive a car: at first it seems impossible to perform and keep in mind all the actions and principles that are required simultaneously. The brain is not good at focusing on more than one thing at a time – and more than three is impossible for most people. However, you focus mostly on a specific action at any particular moment until this starts to become more automatic for you. You can then focus on another simultaneous action until that too becomes automatic. Those two actions now become one, in that they no longer require your full attention, so you can focus on another action. Eventually all the actions become so automatic that they require no conscious effort: driving is just one thing. You can then listen to the radio or have a conversation while driving, something inconceivable in the early stages of learning. The parallel in t'ai chi is being able to add deeper nei gung techniques, one by one, so that what seemed like separate parts become a whole ("separate and then combine"). With this approach, there is no need to feel daunted by the seeming complexity of t'ai chi.

A very useful exercise to help make your form movements more automatic is to practise the entire form without using your arms. Place your hands over your tantien and keep them there, as you run through the form using only your lower body. This will build a solid foundation for all your movements. The t'ai chi classics say: "If there is a

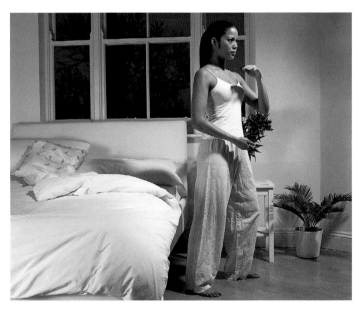

Left Relaxed t'ai chi practice before bedtime can help release nervous tension and prepare you for restful sleep.

Right Shown here is t'ai chi being practised with an emphasis on full awareness of chi flows through the body, and of internal relaxation and development, rather than a concentration on the precision of external movement.

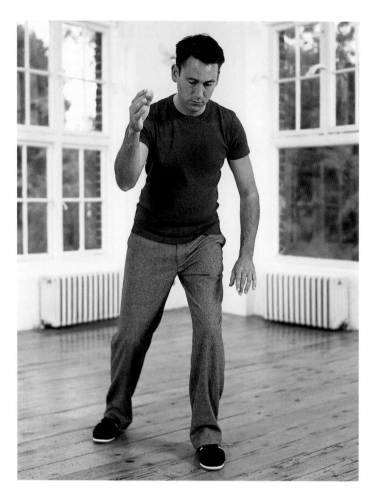

problem, look to the waist and the legs." This means that misalignments and errors in the lower body are usually the cause of errors in the upper body. Most people find it harder to focus on their lower body than on their arms, and training in this way will help correct the situation.

NIGHT AND DAY

New students often ask when is the best time of day to practise t'ai chi. The answer is: whenever they can. Practising first thing in the morning is very beneficial, partly because of the yang energy of that time of day, but if you are too busy then, practise when you can. T'ai chi will not lose its efficacy. Practising last thing at night is also very beneficial as it relaxes your nervous system and releases physical tension before you sleep.

You should not practise when very full or very hungry, though you can practise after a light meal. Practice is not recommended while you are intoxicated, exhausted or ill, as it is best not to manipulate your chi in these circumstances. Men should not practise within one to two hours of sexual activity (orgasm) as their sexual energy needs to restructure without interference. This is less of an issue for women. For women, practising during menstruation, while not harmful, may cause heavier bleeding, as the chi moves or "governs" blood. This could actually be a desirable effect in cases of menstrual cramping, when the blood is not moving freely.

RELAXING INTO YOUR PRACTICE

"Rome wasn't built in a day" – this Western saying is perfectly applicable to t'ai chi and all Taoist self-development practice. Let your practice be a holiday from the pressures of daily life. Ultimately, in t'ai chi there is nothing to achieve: you are simply returning to your natural state, free of your previous tensions. This happens through sustained practice, done without attachment to results. Demanding results of yourself inevitably leads to self-criticism and more tension, and so in the context of t'ai chi practice it is counterproductive. Keep up your regular practice, but relax and, above all, enjoy it. Let t'ai chi become a source of joy in your life, and you will find that your practice naturally develops in ways you never expected.

T'AI CHI THEORY

If you want a better understanding of the theoretical and philosophical underpinnings of t'ai chi, you can study the relationship of the "thirteen postures" of t'ai chi to yin/yang, eight trigram, and Five Element theory. This can lead to insights into the nature of the postures found in t'ai chi and their corresponding energies. It is best undertaken later in

your practice, as you should learn to feel t'ai chi from the beginning, rather than make it an intellectual study. You may also wish to read commentaries on the t'ai chi classics, and commentaries by various t'ai chi masters, for their insights into the theories and methods of practice. This book is intended to give you a foundation in the main principles of t'ai chi, after which you will be better equipped to understand the meanings of the classics and other commentaries, which, if studied at the very beginning of your t'ai chi journey, can be somewhat bewildering, and therefore daunting. Once you have become more familiar with t'ai chi, however, you will find they are more easily understood and very helpful to your continued development.

THE IMPORTANCE OF A TEACHER

This book is intended to give you a good understanding of what t'ai chi is about, and to get you started in your practice. If you follow the exercises in it carefully, you will progress well. However, if you wish to continue with your t'ai chi practice, you should find a competent teacher. Apart from the fact that some techniques are hard to learn without personal guidance, there may be errors in your practice that could be easily corrected with input from a teacher. Additionally, some energetic techniques are best learned directly from a teacher who can perform them themselves. A teacher can guide you to new levels of t'ai chi practice that you would otherwise never even guess existed. This will make you journey into t'ai chi evolve and deepen far beyond your initial expectations.

Deepening Your T'ai Chi Practice

At the heart of t'ai chi lie the methods of Taoist nei gung, and these provide the real benefits of t'ai chi practice. The more nei gung in your t'ai chi, the deeper your practice becomes and the greater the benefits. Some nei gung techniques are harder to master than others, and some offer relatively greater benefits. The best method of progressing is to first learn the movements of the form well, and then start adding nei gung techniques to it.

It is not that some nei gung techniques are more important than others, as ultimately they are synergistic – each aspect of Taoist nei gung helping every other aspect to function fully. However, there are two techniques that can dramatically enhance your t'ai chi practice, in terms of how efficiently you work with your chi, and the degree of energetic and physical releasing that you achieve. These are pulsing and spiralling.

PULSING
Using the technique of pulsing, or "opening and closing", you open and close your joints (and your internal body spaces, such as the kwa) from the inside. This is not the same as bending and folding your limbs at the joints. You cause the space within each joint to change. This is a naturally occurring action, but one that becomes severely diminished as you age. Pulsing not only frees constriction and increases the health of the joints themselves (for instance, increasing the synovial fluid in the joints), but also enables you to gather and release chi very strongly. This in turn releases blockages in the joints, which are the major energetic gates of your body. (The spine is added to this process eventually, using a more advanced nei gung practice known as "bend the bow and shoot the arrow".)

PULSING WITH A PARTNER
If this is done correctly and gently, your wrist will relax substantially and you will feel a greater sense of chi moving through your wrist, hand and arm, in coordination with the pulsing. This will improve your t'ai chi practice.

1 Holding your forearm fixed with one hand, your partner uses the other to pull your hand gently outwards, increasing the space in (and therefore opening) your wrist joint.

2 Your partner returns the joint space to "normal".

3 Your partner gently pushes your hand towards your forearm, decreasing the space in (closing) your wrist joint. When they have found 100 per cent of your range of movement in both directions, they should open and close (pulse) your wrist joint rhythmically, keeping to 70 per cent of that range. Repeat with the other wrist.

T'AI CHI RULER
This exercise allows you to develop joint pulsing within yourself. It is best practised immediately after you have had your joints pulsed by a partner.

Stand normally, arms and legs slightly bent, and bring your hands to about waist height. Open your arms and legs as you stand higher, and allow your hands to move out and up in a circular motion to about shoulder height. As you open up, feel your wrist joints opening internally. Bring your hands back towards you and down to starting position, continuing the circular motion, and bending your arms and legs. As your hands come inwards, feel your wrist joints closing internally. Repeat without stopping, finding your natural rhythm. If you achieve pulsing in your wrist joints, let it spread to your finger joints, then progressively along your arms, through your body and into your legs, until you feel all

Below Pulsing the wrist joint. Here the wrist is shown at its most open point. The next action is to release the pulling open, and then to push inwards, closing the joint. Note the forearm is held fixed.

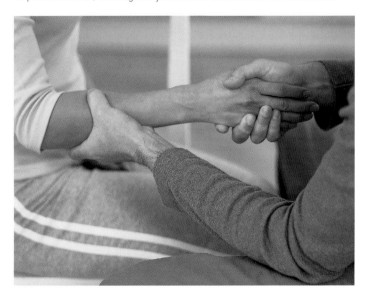

Right This is the most open stage of the t'ai chi ruler exercise. From this point the arms and legs bend as your hands come towards your body. Try to open and close your hands from the centre of the palm (laogung) as you move outwards and inwards.

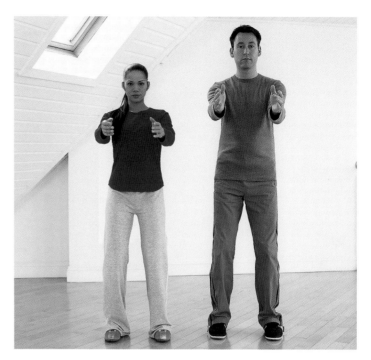

your joints pulsing in coordination, opening and closing with your movements. Feel as if you are drawing energy inwards through your hands on the closings, and releasing energy outwards on the openings. You can then apply opening and closing to the outward and inward actions of the form.

SPIRALLING

The actions of spiralling activate the naturally spiralling flows of chi within you. They also free your muscles, fascia and ligaments, increase blood flow within your tissues, and help your internal organs to move naturally. Once you have a clear understanding of spiralling in your arms and legs, you can combine it with pulsing of the joints, to maximize your energetic work and physical releasing. This will be easier to achieve in Cloud Hands practice (closing as you move towards the centre, opening as you move to either side) than during t'ai chi form practice, but once you have a clear sense of it, you will find it starts to occur naturally in your t'ai chi form. A good teacher can provide further instruction on pulsing and spiralling in t'ai chi.

As you slowly perform Cloud Hands, have your partner help you spiral the tissues of your arms (one arm at a time) in the same direction as the turning of your hands. You should feel your muscles and ligaments twisting around your bones, rather than the bones themselves being twisted by your partner.

While practising Cloud Hands, have a partner spiral the tissues of your legs (one leg at a time) in the same direction as your turn. You should feel your muscles and ligaments twisting around your bones, rather than the bones themselves being twisted. Your partner should spiral the tissues first in your lower legs, and then in your upper legs. With two partners, your lower and upper legs on one side can be spiralled simultaneously, and then both legs can be spiralled at the same time (at the same level). Feel as if the spiralling of your tissues around the bones generates your turn. Your knees should never be twisted in any way. Always exercise caution when spiralling your legs – keep to 70 per cent of your limit, and do not allow your joints to twist.

Below Spiralling the tissues of the arm as it rises in Cloud Hands. Note that the elbow remains dropped, pointing downwards.

Below Spiralling the legs in Cloud Hands. It is vital that the knee joint is not twisted at all – only the muscles of the leg should twist.

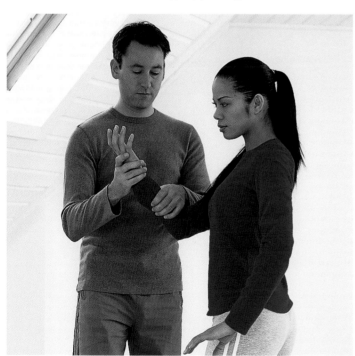

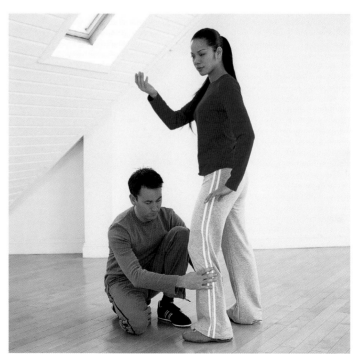

Being Creative – T'ai Chi as an Art

T'ai chi training starts as a science, with many precise principles to learn and apply, but once the science is assimilated, it becomes an art. It can be compared to learning painting techniques or musical theory, and then using those skills to paint or compose freely, applying them in a harmonious and creative way. Advanced principles of t'ai chi – nei gung techniques – are accessed by approaching your practice with a creative mentality.

The creative mind is a natural gift that can become blocked by tensions and fixed ideas about what is possible and how things should be achieved. When you enter your deeper, creative mind, the answers manifest themselves spontaneously. The way you enter this deeper mind is by relaxing and letting go of the desire for specific results, opening yourself to whatever may occur. This is a very important aspect of intermediate and advanced t'ai chi practice.

ADVANCED T'AI CHI PRACTICE

As you become familiar with the form and the main principles of t'ai chi, additional practice methods will help you develop. One of these is to use t'ai chi form postures as standing postures. This means holding a posture for some time (anything between a few minutes and an hour) in order to allow your body to release in that posture and your chi to develop. This can be a painful experience, as you start to feel existing tensions within your body. However, it is a very fast and effective method of releasing those tensions. As a starting point, try standing in the "single whip" posture, and

Below The "single whip" posture is ideal for standing practice. As you stand, maintain your external structure but relax internally.

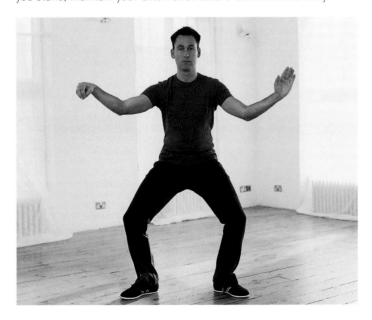

also in the "yin release" posture. Both these positions will help develop your chi and release tension in ways that will benefit you generally. Another useful method is to do your form with your eyes closed. We normally use vision to help with our spatial awareness and balance. Doing t'ai chi with your eyes shut will develop your balance and physical awareness and help you find your internal stability.

RIGHT- AND LEFT-HANDED FORMS

All t'ai chi forms are "handed", meaning that the movements and postures are not symmetrical: you will work one side of your body comparatively more than the other. Normally, you will learn a right-handed form to start with. You should train with this for approximately three years before learning to perform an exact mirror image of the form. After this, you may choose to perform both equally, or to emphasize either the left- or right-handed form to open up that side of your body. If you choose the latter, you would practise a ratio of at least 2:1 on the side you want to work on. It is important that you become very confident with the initial, right-handed form before attempting a left-handed form. If you are genuinely left-handed (rather than only writing with your left hand) you may want to reverse the order and start with a left-handed form, in which case you should seek the guidance of a teacher.

Most people have imbalances between the left and right sides of their body. One side will be more tense or blocked, energetically and/or physically. You should always play to your weaker side, moving only as much on your stronger side as you can on the weaker side. This way, your weaker side will draw energy from your stronger, and will improve, rather than the opposite. This principle also applies when doing a moving chi gung such as Cloud Hands.

NEI GUNG TECHNIQUES

T'ai chi is principally about implementing Taoist nei gung principles within yourself. The form exists to help you do this in an efficient way (as well as having martial functions). The physical movements of the form are not t'ai chi. They are what an untrained observer will see as t'ai chi, but as

Right Playing with the form. Although the movements may not correspond to specific postures in the form, all the t'ai chi principles of alignment and movement are present. As you learn nei gung methods this can be a powerful way of developing these techniques in a freer, more spontaneous way.

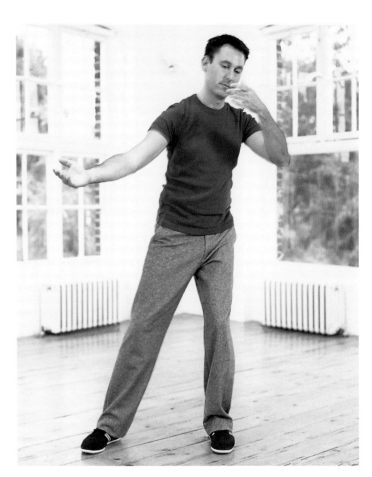

you progress you will come to realize that t'ai chi is really what is going on within you. This is, of course, all but invisible to the average outside observer.

Every posture in the form has several variations; some relate to your level of practice, others are simply different ways of performing a technique. Nothing is written in stone apart from the fundamental, underlying principles of t'ai chi. Once you are very familiar with the form, you will start to work on various nei gung techniques, adding them to your form practice one by one. Pulsing and spiralling are two very important examples, but there are many others. They include the stretching and release of the ligaments, which also brings about strong emotional release; the movement of the fascial tissues and chi in wavelike motions up and down the body, activating the yin and yang meridians; the "wrapping of tissues" from the back of the body to the front and vice versa, activating horizontal flows of chi; the deliberate movement of the fluids of the body; the incorporation of circles and spirals into all your movements; the movement of energy both up and down in the body, and from centre to periphery and back again; and the movement of energy into and out of the spine and tantien.

FREEING YOUR FORM
As you continue with your t'ai chi form practice, you might find that your experience of it becomes a little rigid and lacking in spontaneity. Ultimately, spontaneity in practice comes from what is happening within your body. In order to break free of any feeling of rigidity it can be very useful, and enjoyable, to "play" with the form.

A good starting point for this is "drunken" t'ai chi. In this method of practice, your main focus is on completely releasing the nervous system, including the brain. As you run through your form at a slow pace, allow your nervous system to relax and release as completely as possible. The result will be movement that flops and jiggles as you release tensions in your nerves. If you succeed in releasing tension in the brain as well, you will find that your eyelids flutter. Allow yourself to stagger and lose balance, if that occurs spontaneously. Do not give any thought to t'ai chi principles or being "correct" in your form. This method is extremely relaxing and very useful if you are stressed and holding nervous tension. It is especially beneficial when practised immediately before going to sleep.

SPONTANEOUS MOVEMENT
Once you have learned to relax your nervous system through "drunken" t'ai chi, you can start to play with your t'ai chi form. At first, try varying the movements: see if you can

alter a movement while retaining a sense of flow and adhering to t'ai chi principles. Try making your movements more circular, even if this means doing an "incorrect" move. Try to get the circles you are doing with your arms to spread into your shoulder blades, moving and releasing these "hidden joints of the body". Take the circles and spirals into all parts of your body, especially parts that feel stuck or relatively lifeless, to wake up and release those areas. Eventually, try not only to take the circles and spirals to your lower tantien, but to make them originate from it, and spread to all parts of your body. In t'ai chi, all movement, both energetic and physical, originates in the tantien.

At this point in your practice, you may find that you are doing "spontaneous" movements that allow you to carry out this internal work, and no longer doing a t'ai chi form. Continue with this, being creative and letting your body show you how you can manifest these circles and spirals. Now be conscious of your alignments, and, as you move, be aware of when your body feels open and correctly aligned, and when it closes down. Learn from this with an open mind. Play with these alignments, and find what works best for you. Be conscious of gathering and releasing energy as you move, in an alternating, pulsating way. Let your chi move out from your centre (tantien and spine) and back again. Find which sort of rhythm enhances this.

After you have practised in this spontaneous way, go back to your form practice, relaxing and observing any changes in the way your form feels. It should feel freer and more alive. You will have gained a much greater understanding of some of the nei gung principles of t'ai chi.

Exercises for Meditation

The following exercises will help you explore meditation practice more deeply and start to integrate it with your t'ai chi practice. They mainly involve using your awareness of your breath in order to lead your mind inwards and release tensions on your emotional level (although your mental and psychic energies may also be accessed). Sitting meditation is an excellent adjunct to t'ai chi, both before and after practising the form.

Your breath is the most direct link between your mind (awareness) and your energy, whether physical (chi) or emotional. Using breathing meditation techniques, you can connect with progressively deeper levels of your energy. Initially, you might feel slightly more nervous, but this means that your awareness is going deeper and you are noticing internal tensions that already exist. Persevere, and these tensions will dissolve.

FOLLOWING THE BREATH

Sitting comfortably, follow your breath progressively down your central channel to your lower tantien, as in Taoist breathing practice. However, this time focus more on your emotional (and mental, and psychic) energies as you breathe. Throughout your downward progression be especially aware of the quality of your breath – whether the breath itself is smooth and "neutral", or whether it contains some vibration, charge, tension or agitation, however subtle.

Anything in your breath that is not completely smooth is an indication of internal tension, most often in your emotional energy. The breath is the principal medium whereby emotional tension can release; it is also the principal means by which you can become more aware of emotional tension. Let your breath be the guide to your deeper emotional states, and let it be the means to you becoming emotionally "smooth". Allow any tension or vibration in your breath to release of its own accord as you breathe out. Use your in-breath to become aware of emotional tension (within your breath), and your out-breath to allow it to release, by relaxing the breath itself and letting it become smooth and "empty". Continue this process as you follow your breath down your central channel. If you experience any sort of vibration, charge or sensation in the breath (or in any part of yourself) that you find impossible to understand – because it does not seem to relate to any form of emotion or anything you can "identify" – this may mean that you have encountered blockage or tension in your psychic energy. In any case, apply the same method of allowing your breath to become smooth as you breathe out,

Below Breathing meditation practised lying down allows for greater physical relaxation. Make sure your awareness remains focused.

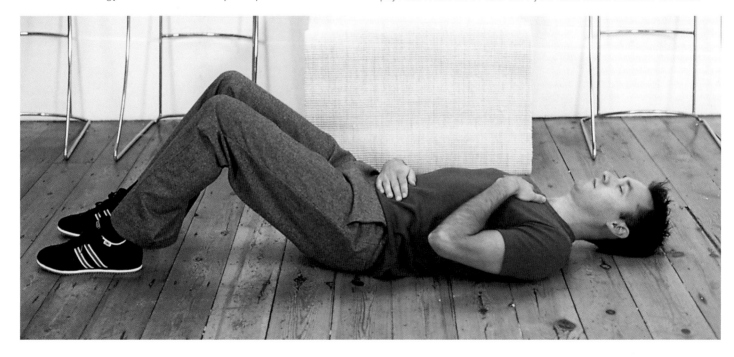

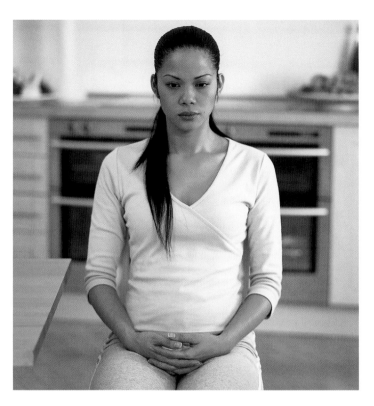

Above Meditation with the eyes open. Taoist practices combine internal (nei) with external (wei) awareness. Sitting meditation is an excellent starting point for this.

in order to release that tension. Throughout this practice, adopt an attitude of being willing to experience whatever "comes up" while you are practising, with the knowledge that whatever is inside you must be experienced fully in order for it to be released fully.

MEDITATION WITH EYES OPEN

Once you feel comfortable with this method of breathing meditation, practise with your eyes open, keeping them very relaxed and neutral. Allow the images of your surroundings to come into you, through your eyes, rather than projecting your mind outward through your eyes. Maintain full awareness internally, while simultaneously being aware of your surroundings. After practising sitting, with your eyes open, practise standing in the wu chi standing posture, eyes open. Then practise while walking slowly, with full awareness. Following this, practise while doing Cloud Hands chi gung. If you practise the open-eyed method of breathing meditation well, you will find that you can achieve an effortless, relaxed focus in all activities. You will gain a sense of equanimity, regardless of what takes place around you, greatly reducing your stress response to outside events.

T'AI CHI MEDITATION

After you have become familiar with eyes-open practice while sitting, standing, walking and during Cloud Hands, you can apply breathing meditation while performing your form. Avoid correcting your form while practising t'ai chi meditation. Allow yourself to relax fully, letting your body perform the movements automatically while your awareness

is on your breath. Be especially aware of the places where you change from yin to yang and vice versa, both in your physical movements and your breathing.

You may wish to slow your movements down considerably as you approach these yin/yang changeover points, to allow release to occur and to enter deeper levels of stillness. It is at the changeover points that you are most likely to encounter stillness, and release deeply held tension. Allow your form to become naturally smaller and "looser". If you find you need to concentrate on the sequence of movements of the form, practise using only the commencement until your form movements are truly automatic. As a general rule, the more slowly you move the deeper your awareness will go, allowing for deeper release. Adopt a gradual approach to slowing your practice speed; experiencing and releasing emotional tension can be an intense experience – stay within the comfort zone.

Below Practising t'ai chi form for meditation. Note that the body and limbs are looser and the posture smaller than in normal form practice. Total release of tension is the goal.

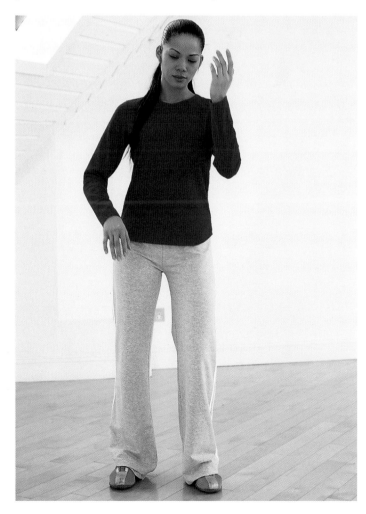

Push Hands

Tui shou (push hands) training is indispensable for furthering your t'ai chi practice. It also forms the bridge to the practice of t'ai chi as a martial art. However, it is not a martial practice in itself, and should be used even if you have no interest in the martial aspects of t'ai chi. Done correctly, it embodies the t'ai chi philosophy of relaxation, yielding, sensitivity and appropriateness of action.

Its benefits derive mainly from the fact that in push hands practice you are working with a partner, in a way that can be either cooperative or challenging. The interplay of chi between push hands partners allows for very efficient release of chi blockages in both practitioners.

BASIC PRINCIPLES

As you practise push hands exercises, try to remain as relaxed as possible. Adopt the attitude that even if your partner is trying to push you, this is by mutual consent, and is in order to help you develop your skills. Be aware of any emotional response that the exercises evoke, and try to relax that. Push hands is not sparring, and should not be practised with any "hard" martial intent, or you will not benefit from it fully. If you have an interest in t'ai chi as a martial art, the relaxation under pressure that you gain from push hands will form a foundation for t'ai chi fighting.

Retain all the key t'ai chi alignment and movement principles as you go through these exercises. Try to use a minimum of physical strength and maintain contact at all times, "listening" to your partner's movement and chi and not opposing it. Maintain awareness of your breathing: never hold your breath, and allow any emotional tension to release, as in t'ai chi form practice. Bear in mind the principle, "Four

Benefits of push hands
Push hands is important for all t'ai chi practitioners for the following reasons:
- It tests your ability to gain and develop an energetic "root", as well as helping you develop your root.
- It highlights those areas of your body that may be stiff or tense, and allows you to relax them consciously.
- It tests and develops your application of the key t'ai chi principles regarding alignment and movement.
- It provides an environment in which you can become more aware of tension in your nervous system, and allow it to release.
- It highlights emotions such as anger and fear, and allows you to relax and reduce your glandular response to external pressure. In conjunction with meditation practice, it makes you more aware of your ego and your need to win.

ounces can defeat ten thousand pounds," meaning that a very light force applied correctly can divert a very large force, without trying to oppose it. This is like leading a large bull by the ring through its nose – it cannot resist.

PUSH HANDS PRACTICE

As you repeat these exercises, focus on relaxing your nervous system and mind, on rooting, alignments and weight transfer. Ideally, your partner should feel as if they have nothing to push on – like pushing at thin air – and you should feel as if you have used no effort to yield to and divert their force. Neither person should push forward or yield further than correct alignments will allow. When you have finished the following sequence, change legs and arms. You can also practise this exercise with the opposite leg and arm combination as well as turning/diverting inwards rather than outwards.

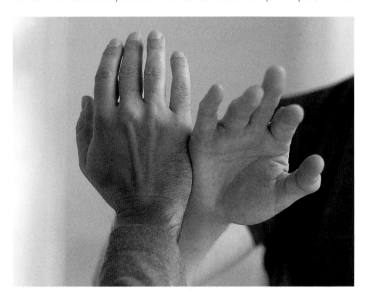

Left Making contact at the wrists. Try to feel as if you are "stuck" to your partner's wrist, always maintaining light and relaxed contact.

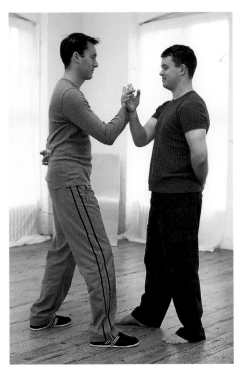

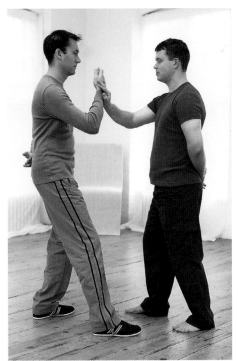

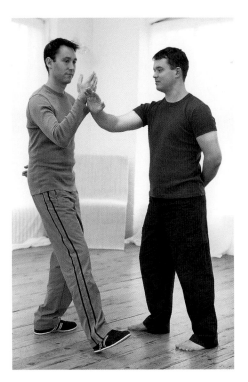

1 Start with both partners adopting the stance shown here, opposing feet stepped towards each other and opposing wrists lightly touching, back to back. Put your other hand in the small of your back.

2 As your partner shifts their weight fully forwards, turning their palm outwards to push the back of your wrist, start to shift your own weight back, yielding to your partner's pressure, but keeping your "courtyard" – the space between your arm and body – intact.

3 As you shift your weight fully to your back leg, turn your centre outwards as shown, keeping your arm connected to your spine and bringing it with the turn. Turn up to 45 degrees, diverting your partner's force away from your centre.

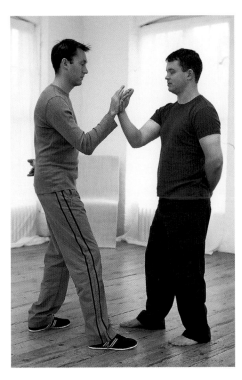

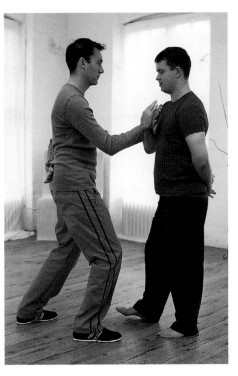

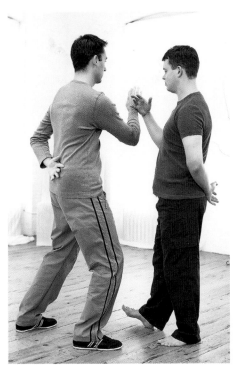

4 As you reach the end of your yielding and diverting movement, start turning back to the centre, turning your palm towards your partner and beginning to push as they turn the back of their wrist towards you.

5 As you return to the centre (facing your partner), start shifting your weight forwards, pushing towards your partner's centre at heart height.

6 As you do this, your partner should yield to and divert your push just as you did theirs. At the end of their movement, they will start pushing back towards you. Repeat the cycle.

Push Hands Training Exercises

The following training exercises will help you develop rooting, yielding/diverting, body and leg alignments, and stability in the upper and lower body. The push should be slow, with force building gradually.

YIELDING AND DIVERTING

These exercises are designed to develop further your ability to remain stable and rooted even while you are being pushed. The force of the push is either yielded to and diverted by turning the spine, or at a more advanced level, is yielded to internally – the energy of the push is allowed to travel unhindered down through the body and into the ground. Your partner will feel as if they are either pushing on thin air, or that they are pushing against the ground.

1 As you stand in a front-weighted stance, your partner pushes slowly on your shoulder. Yield to this force, while maintaining alignments. Repeat on the other side, then change legs and repeat, then do the same with a back-weighted stance.

2 Return to a front-weighted stance while your partner pushes slowly in the centre of your chest. Change legs and repeat, as before, and then do the same with a back-weighted stance.

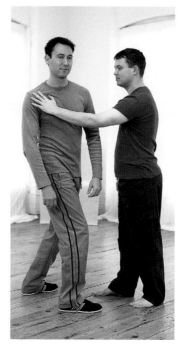
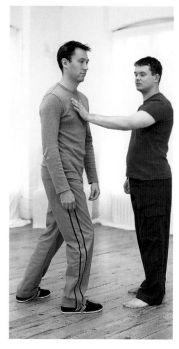

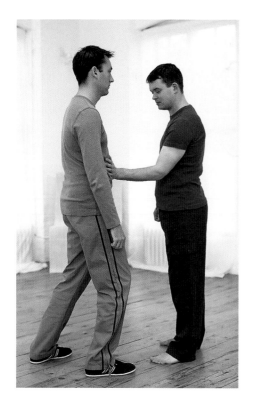
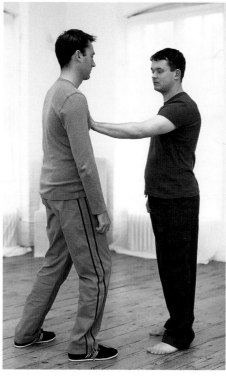
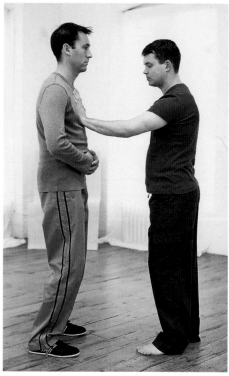

3 Repeat the exercise with your partner pushing on your belly, in the centre just below your ribcage. Once again, change legs and repeat, and then repeat on a back-weighted stance.

4 Starting in a front-weighted stance, have your partner push straight forwards at the centre of your chest. Without shifting weight or diverting the push by turning, try to sink the force of the push downwards through your body and legs into the ground. This is yielding internally (downwards).

5 If this is successful, try standing normally in an even-weighted "wu chi" posture and repeat. Let this exercise help you feel where you are internally bound and blocked: try to relax those places inside your body so the energy of the push can pass through you and drop into the ground.

ROOTING EXERCISES

The following three exercises help you develop your rooting skills and body alignments. Standing in wu chi posture, take a few moments to become as rooted as possible, getting your chi to sink to your tantien and into the ground. Have your partner test your alignments and rooting by pushing gently and slowly (not abruptly) at the sides of your body, arms, legs and even your head, one side at a time. You will easily feel where your alignments are correct and it requires no effort to resist the push (other than the basic energy required to maintain your structure), and where your body "jams up" and you need real effort to resist a push. Adjust your alignments at those places and retest the posture. In a more advanced practice, using your intent, try to bring your chi to the site of the push, minimizing the physical effort needed to resist. Repeat the previous exercise with pushes

Below The posture "double an" from the "grasp sparrow's tail" sequence of the t'ai chi form, being tested by a partner.

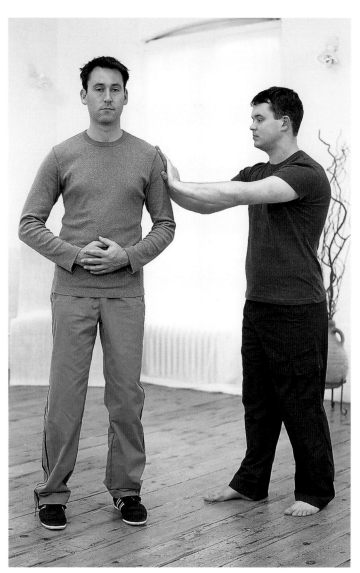

Above Rooting exercises basically test how secure your stance is, and whether your body is aligned correctly.

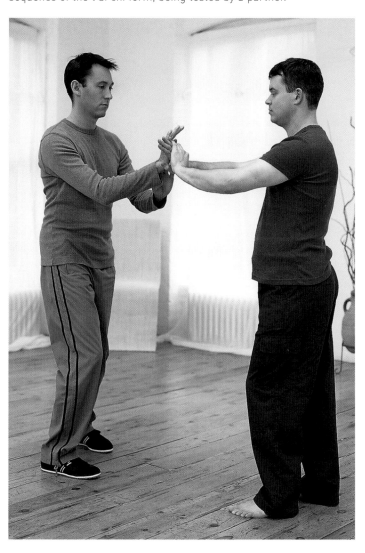

on the front and back of your body. Once you are comfortable with these exercises, have your partner gently push randomly on any part of the body, at any angle. You will find that some of the angles will naturally be harder to resist than others.

Assume a posture from the t'ai chi form, and have your partner test it by pushing and pulling on you from various angles. This type of static posture testing is very important in t'ai chi as a means of discovering the precise body alignments that allow your chi to flow fully in each posture. By doing this you will also discover the relative strengths and weaknesses of each posture in the form, and better understand the characteristic energies of each posture.

When you do this posture testing you will find that if your arms are overextended or too withdrawn, the posture is weak – in other words, your chi is not flowing strongly. What you are seeking is an ideal balance of yin and yang within each posture, which gives it a natural and effortless strength, both structurally and energetically. Understanding the nature of each posture will greatly help you understand t'ai chi in all its forms and principles.

Push Hands Variations

The single push hands exercise is the foundation of push hands practice. Once the basic skills have been developed you may wish to learn other variations, such as double push hands, and push hands at different heights, such as high push hands and low push hands.

These advanced push hands exercises train different parts of the body and develop different forms of yielding, diverting and pushing, as well as helping you to release different parts of your body. Martially, they train your awareness and movement skills at different heights and in response to a variety of potential techniques an opponent might employ.

One of the key skills that push hands training develops is that of "ting jin" (listening energy). This involves being sensitive to your partner's movement, energy and even mental intent so that you react appropriately to their actions, always one step ahead of them. This ability to be sensitive to and interpret other people's intentions, and then act appropriately and with perfect timing, is a very useful skill in many areas of life outside of t'ai chi practice. Once you have developed your "listening" skills, you can develop your "jan" (yielding), "lan" (merging) and "nien" (adhering) skills. The highest level of this progression is "suei" (magnetizing), but this is a very rare skill indeed.

FA JIN

Fa means "issuing", and jin means "power", and "fa jin" relates to the fast release of energy, in order to uproot, move and/or strike an opponent. It can also be used in healing practice (such as chi gung tui na, or massage) to clear energetic blockages in a patient. In the context of t'ai chi practice, and specifically push hands, it is used to push a partner/opponent away from you. It can also be used to clear chi stagnation from your or your partner's body.

There are many levels of skill in "fa jin". The highest levels rely almost solely on chi projection, rather than biomechanical action (such as joint compression/release

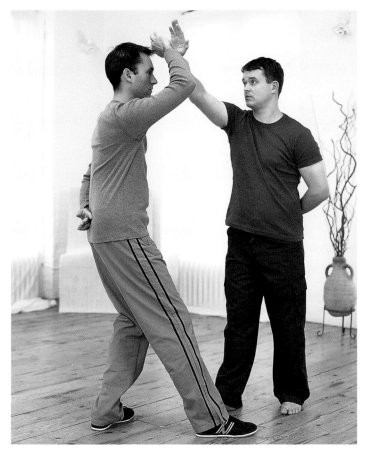

Above High push hands. As your partner pushes towards your head, shift your weight back and yield and divert upwards and out.

and ligament release). At a very high level, fa jin seems mysterious when experienced. It can feel as if you are being picked up and moved a large distance as if by a wind, with no real force having been applied to you. Use the squat and tuck that you have learned already to develop your gathering and release skills. Do not tense or "push" as you release – simply let go outwards, and fa jin will start to occur.

VARIATIONS

T'ai chi push hands uses specific training methods to develop your skill in relation to different areas of the body and (with a view to martial skill) in relation to different techniques you might encounter. Double push hands develops the ability to coordinate both hands in relation to a double-handed push or technique from your partner. The specifics of this method need to be learned from a teacher. High push hands relates to a push or strike aimed at the head, and helps you remain "dropped" and relaxed while raising your arms. Similarly there are low push hands training methods, relating to the lower body, as well as specific variations dealing with other angles.

Below Double push hands in the Wu style. This is a set sequence of actions that manifests "peng", "lu", "ji" and "an" energy in sequence.

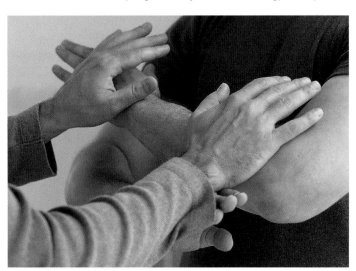

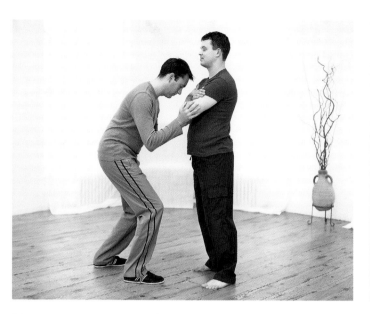

Above Gathering chi energy (including your partner's chi) as you squat in preparation for issuing in "fa jin".

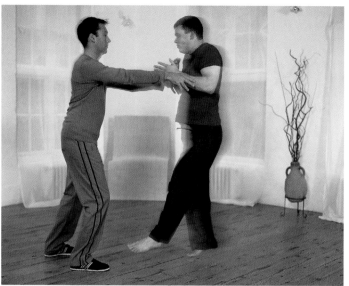

Above Tucking the tailbone and standing up as you release gathered chi rapidly with "fa jin". Note that the partner has become uprooted.

CIRCLING HANDS

This freer, more spontaneous form of push hands can provide a transition into t'ai chi sparring (martial practice). The use of circles is strongly emphasized: your arms and those of your partner circle continuously, touching at the wrist. These circles are mirrored in your body, eventually originating from within your lower tantien as internal movements that cause external circles to manifest.

At first, circling hands should be practised with a view to developing listening energy in relation to your partner's movements, and using circular movement to release your body. Once you have established a relaxed rhythm, you can try pushing your opponent when an opportunity presents itself. You can push on any part of your partner's body, at any angle. Find out by trial and error what does and does not work, in terms of both timing and technique. Aggressive,

rapid pushing is not required if you use good timing and judgement. Try to maintain a flow, even when you attempt to push. If your partner attempts to push you, use circularity of movement and the skills you have gained so far to yield and divert their force.

As a transition into t'ai chi sparring, you can also attempt to slap your partner (gently) at various places on the body, rather than just pushing. You can also apply t'ai chi techniques such as "shoulder stroke", "elbow strike", "split" and "pull down". It is a good idea to discuss the rules of this practice before you begin, to establish whether you both consent to pushing, gentle slaps or harder contact, so that neither of you will feel aggrieved if you are on the receiving end of a push or slap. You are engaging in this practice to help each other develop, not to make enemies, or hurt each other. Try to stay relaxed, whatever happens.

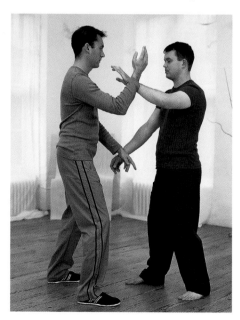

1 For circling hands, stand as shown and circle your hands, wrists touching.

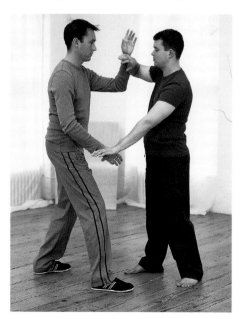

2 Shift your weight and turn your body as appropriate.

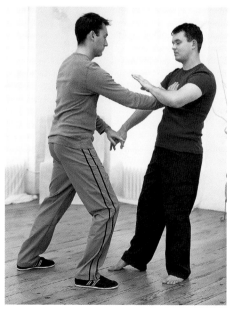

3 Open your partner's centre with the left hand and push with the right.

T'ai Chi as a Martial Art

Though t'ai chi chuan is a practical martial art, the vast majority of people who practise it today do so for its benefits in health and stress reduction, rather than as a self-defence or fighting practice. T'ai chi does not yield martial ability easily – it requires prolonged and intensive practice to become a proficient t'ai chi fighter. This is because it requires development of Taoist nei gung skills in order to fight without using any tension or anger.

From a purely martial perspective, the benefits of this method of fighting are greater awareness, responsiveness, appropriateness of action and power. These skills grow over the years, as opposed to waning with age – a common problem for external martial artists.

EXTERNAL AND INTERNAL

The external martial arts are so-called because they do not use internal, nei gung principles. Instead they rely on muscular strength, speed and aggression. Most popular martial arts are of this type, such as karate, jujitsu, taekwondo, Thai/kick-boxing and kung fu. Interestingly, Western boxing adopts a more relaxed and circular fighting method than many of the Oriental external martial arts. The development of strength, speed and aggression can make you a very good fighter, sometimes in a relatively short time (depending on your ability). However, there are several disadvantages to this type of training: regular practice involving the deliberate use of aggression (anger) does not allow for the smooth release of this type of emotion. On the contrary, it tends to power-up existing emotions within you,

which is not helpful for your personal development. Physical tension is not released, and may even increase as a result of training. Damage may be inflicted on the body (especially the joints) over time, which can lead to problems such as arthritis later in life. These factors depend on the severity of your training regime, but in order to become a "serious" martial artist, you must train hard. Almost none of the deeper self-development benefits of the internal martial arts are gained with external martial arts training.

If you genuinely feel the need to defend yourself against aggression, an external martial art may provide the answer. If not, then you would benefit from examining your motivation for wanting to practise a martial art. If it is principally for self-development, an internal martial art such as t'ai chi may be ideal. When practised correctly it can make you more relaxed, healthier and more emotionally balanced as you age, and, in time, a proficient martial artist.

Below A classic image of external martial arts: power, speed and aggression are being used to overwhelm the opponent in this women's taekwondo competition.

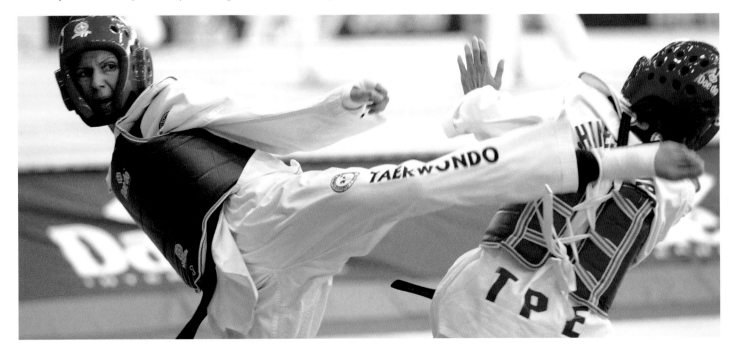

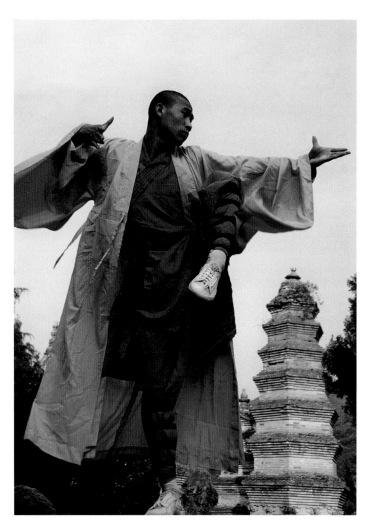

Right A Chinese Shaolin monk practising kung fu. There are chi development practices in Shaolin styles but they do not adhere to the t'ai chi principles of relaxation. External, muscular strength and tension are deliberately employed to generate power.

KUNG FU

Most of the kung fu style martial arts do not share any of the core principles of t'ai chi chuan, hsing-i chuan or ba gua zhang. Kung fu (pronounced "gung fu") means "work" (or "effort") and "time" – in other words, skill gained from prolonged practice. The phrase can be applied to any activity, from that of a chef or a carpenter to a martial artist. A better term is "wushu" (fighting method). There are many highly developed and colourful "wushu" styles in existence, such as "praying mantis". These are effective martial arts but they use external principles and training methods, and should not be confused with the internal martial arts simply because of their Chinese origins. Semi-internal or external/ internal Chinese styles also exist, such as "monkey boxing" and "eight drunken immortals". These are closer to the internal styles but still use some external training methods and principles.

T'AI CHI FIGHTING

Push hands and circling hands practice forms a bridge to martial t'ai chi practice, as it develops your ability to root, relax under pressure, interpret and respond to an opponent, understand fighting angles and use them to your advantage, and issue power. Less obvious is how t'ai chi form practice relates to real-life fighting.

The slowness of t'ai chi form practice allows for the release of tensions at every level – especially of the nervous system. The limiting factor on speed of movement is tension in the nervous system. When the nerves relax, not only do the muscles relax, but nerve signals can flow more freely and rapidly. This allows for much faster movement when fighting. T'ai chi masters are known for possessing extraordinary speed of movement, being able to change from one technique to the next with lightning speed. This ability is enhanced by the use of circles in movement, and circularity of thinking – not becoming mentally "stuck" at any moment. The greater awareness that t'ai chi practice brings – a truly relaxed focus – allows for the exploitation of an opponent's mental "gaps". You do not gap, or do so significantly less than your opponent. The exploitation of these gaps – moments when someone loses awareness of what is happening – is a major factor in high-level martial arts of any kind. A boxer who says, "I didn't see it coming," has been hit while he was gapping. Some t'ai chi masters can directly (psychically) induce an opponent to gap.

T'ai chi form postures and movements programme various martial techniques into your system, which can then emerge spontaneously during sparring or fighting. These techniques, whether throws, kicks or strikes, can be further developed while sparring with a partner. The sequence of techniques – indeed the techniques themselves – used in the form do not imply that you would use exactly those techniques while fighting. T'ai chi is about principles, and at an intermediate and higher level t'ai chi fighting is extraordinarily spontaneous, the only rule being that the key principles are maintained.

The use of chi energy is central to t'ai chi strikes and kicks – using the same external technique, this energy can be focused either to move an opponent harmlessly or to cause serious internal injury. The amount of power generated by a true internal strike far exceeds that from any "external" strike, and has to be experienced to be believed.

T'ai chi fighters make use of the principle, "start after your opponent, arrive before him". This skill has been likened to the way a cat waits until after a mouse starts to run, and then intercepts it further along its trajectory. It is initially developed through push hands practice. A good t'ai chi fighter always seems to be at least one step ahead of their opponent. Additionally, the saying, "give your opponent what they want, but not the way they expect it," means not opposing them head-on, but luring them into a trap. "Forget yourself and follow the other" applies here (and in push hands), where the "other" is your partner or opponent. T'ai chi fighting skills can seem mysterious to the uninitiated – almost supernatural – but in reality they are abilities that most people can develop, with sufficient application.

FIGHTING WITHOUT ANGER

Assuming that you are not expecting to need to defend yourself against a physical attack, you might ask why you should be interested in practising t'ai chi as a martial art. From the point of view of advancing your t'ai chi practice in general, martial training can provide a clear test of your development. Martial practice gives you a greater understanding of your t'ai chi form practice in terms of the chi movements and transformations that take place in it.

FIGHT OR FLIGHT

The principal benefit of martial training lies in developing the ability to remain calm under extreme pressure. There is arguably no greater stress-causing event than having a person try to hurt you physically. Naturally, you would not train to this extreme under normal circumstances. Sparring would not be escalated to the point where your opponent was genuinely trying to cause you injury unless you were training for real life-or-death conflict, in which case the realism of an all-out attack would be an essential part of your training. Nevertheless, having a sparring partner attempting to make even light contact will almost certainly

Below Responding to a punch with yielding, turning and sticking, simultaneously applying a joint lock/break, while remaining centred.

trigger your natural fear response (often known as "fight or flight"). The moment this response is triggered, your adrenal glands "fire up", secreting large amounts of adrenalin. Your vision narrows, your heart beats rapidly, your breathing becomes shallow and rapid and your nervous system becomes over-stimulated, resulting in physical tension. At the emotional level, a common response to the fear stimulus is anger. This fear/anger response is deliberately utilized in the external martial arts. One of the reasons that the internal martial arts are superior from a fighting perspective is that this adrenalin response actually limits speed of movement and perception (even though it does provide an initial "boost"). The relaxed and open mental awareness and relaxed, powerful and quick movements of a good internal practitioner provide an edge when fighting a "fired-up" external practitioner.

The fight or flight response sets in motion a set of bodily responses that can lead to a number of serious stress-related diseases. Even a moderate triggering of this response, when repeated regularly, will degrade your health, and many events in daily life can cause it. Adrenalin is secreted quickly, but only eliminated slowly from the body. Your system needs sufficient time between stressful events to reduce your adrenalin levels. The constant secretion of adrenalin will keep your body in semi-permanent stress

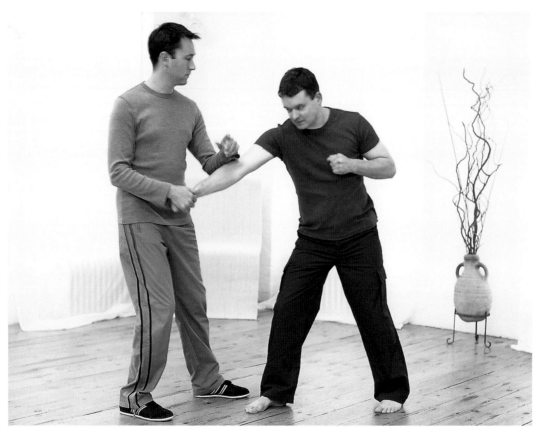

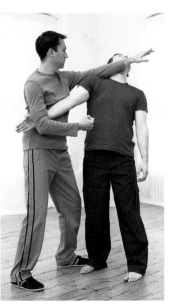

Below Following up by trapping the opponent's arm and using the body to apply a lock/break while attacking the opponent's throat and taking his balance. From here he could easily be thrown backwards.

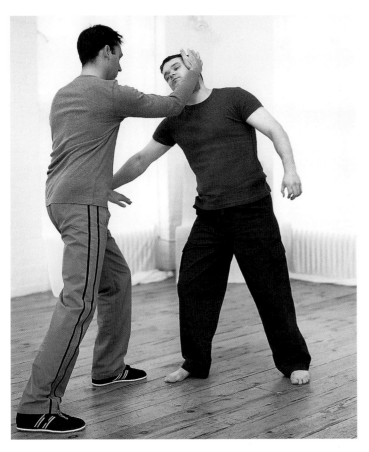

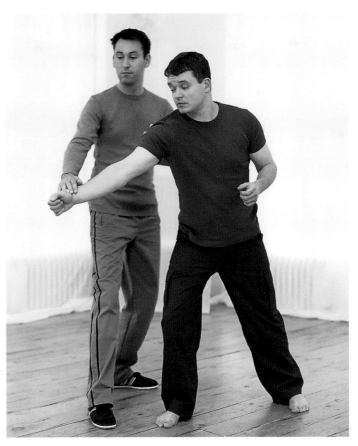

Above Brushing away (diverting) an attack and simultaneously striking the side of the opponent's head. Note his balance has been taken. T'ai chi specializes in swift counter-attacking techniques.

Above Moving swiftly to step to the side of an attacker and subtly control his arm. This would be especially appropriate if he was armed with a knife. He is now very vulnerable to attack from behind.

mode, exhaust your adrenal glands, and from a Chinese medical viewpoint, will deplete your kidney energy (your core energy). Adrenalin can also be addictive, leading you to seek out stressful situations or stimuli, despite the negative effects on your physical and mental health.

During t'ai chi martial training you learn to relax the adrenal response, under the pressure of your training partner's attacks, by using techniques such as releasing emotional tension through the breath, and relaxing nervous system tension as it occurs. In this respect, t'ai chi sparring is an extension of the work you do in push hands practice. The result is that you are able to remain free of the fight or flight stress response even in "stressful" situations. Not only does this benefit your health, but it makes it more likely that your reaction to everyday situations will be calm, measured and appropriate, and that you will not respond in ways that you might later regret.

FIGHTING AND MEDITATION

T'ai chi martial training brings up latent, deeply hidden emotional tensions, often in the form of fear or anger. Once recognized, they can be released during meditation practice. Sometimes, a t'ai chi martial practitioner who is also a meditation practitioner will stop sparring or training when they experience these emotions, and practise sitting meditation for a while in order to release the emotion, before going back to sparring.

After you have practised meditation for some time, you will find that because you have released many of your more surface-level tensions, what remains is deeper, more hidden and harder to identify. Martial training can help you find where these deep tensions lie. Ultimately, martial training confronts you with your own ego, and is in many ways a short cut, albeit a challenging one, to accessing this level of meditation practice.

SELF-DEFENCE

Although your main motivation for martial practice may be its self-development aspects, there is the added benefit of gaining self-defence skills. This is particularly suitable for women, as t'ai chi does not rely on muscular strength, an area where many women are at a disadvantage. The development of internal power can give a woman the ability to defend herself against a physically stronger attacker. There have been many proficient female t'ai chi fighters throughout China's history. T'ai chi martial training gives many women a very welcome sense of self-confidence in relation to their physical safety. Additionally, it can help anybody respond appropriately in physically challenging situations – for instance, you may simply want to restrain or control a person who does not have truly malicious intent. You will have the presence of mind and confidence in your ability to use much less force than you would need to if someone was trying to cause you serious harm.

The T'ai Chi Lifestyle

T'ai chi is very much about achieving balance on every level of your being – physical, energetic, mental and emotional. This philosophy of balance can be extended to encompass all aspects of your life, from the moment you wake in the morning to the time you go to sleep. Since t'ai chi is more than just a specific practice that you do for a set time every day it can become an invaluable guide to leading a healthier, more balanced life.

The principles that you learn and practise in your t'ai chi form and push hands sessions can be applied generally, sometimes with dramatically positive results. If you re-examine your lifestyle, behaviour and habits in the light of your t'ai chi knowledge, you can see where imbalances exist, and their consequences. This can cause you to re-evaluate certain long-term habits and attitudes, and bring about positive change in those areas of your life that you may have found less than satisfactory. Just as in your t'ai chi form practice you seek to balance the releasing and gathering of energy, so there should be a balance between these two in other areas of your life. Naturally, change will occur only if you want it to – your intention is everything.

WORK AND MONEY

One of the major areas of your life that can become a cause of imbalance, and even ill health, is that of work. Most people need to work to earn a living, and in fact work can give you a sense of purpose and direction, self-worth and achievement. Work can be seen as a yang activity, just as resting can be seen as yin. It is appropriate to have a balance of the two: all rest and no work can result in stagnation of your energy. Work involves an expenditure of energy, whether physical or mental, and resting involves the replenishing of energy. Work is probably the greatest expenditure of energy in your life, and your approach to it is a major factor in leading a balanced life.

If you overwork, you expend more energy than you replenish (this could be said to be the definition of overwork) and, just like spending more than you earn, you end up in debt. In this case the debt is energetic, and in order to settle it you have to tap into your deepest reserves – your pre-birth jing. This is like selling the family silver: once it is gone, it is gone for ever. The longer you sustain this level of overwork, the greater the problem. In Taoist terms, the only valid reason for depleting your essence is if your life immediately depends on it: for instance if you are stuck on a mountain freezing in a blizzard. If you are tapping into this essence for any other reason, you have to re-evaluate those aspects of your life that are causing you to do so.

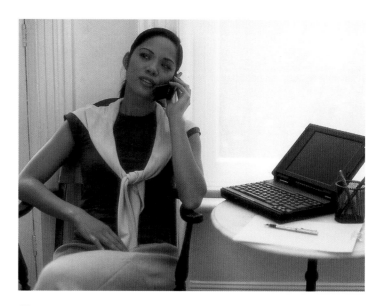

Above Work is an essential part of life, but it must be balanced with the need for rest and recreation if we are to truly enjoy our lives. Material desires can often distort this balance.

Some people overwork because they have genuinely difficult lives – they may be struggling to support a large family – but many others overwork for less critical reasons, such as excessive ambition or in order to sustain a luxurious lifestyle. This is not to say there is anything wrong with wanting physical comforts and luxuries, but from a Taoist perspective to pursue these at the expense of health and mental/emotional well-being is an unbalanced attitude. Any attitudes or habits that seriously threaten your health should be carefully examined. It is essential to find a balance between the desire for money and a successful career, and the maintenance of mental and physical health. Where this balance lies varies from person to person, but the principle can be very useful in finding it for yourself.

CONFLICT

Mental and emotional stress does not come only from overwork. Your home life might be a major cause of stress, resulting from bringing up children, dealing with partners and lovers, friends, parents and relations. Often these

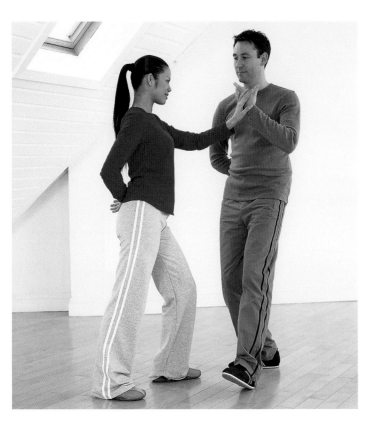

Left The principles of push hands embody the core philosophy of t'ai chi and can teach you to lead a more harmonious emotional life both at work and at home.

issues can be less clear-cut and harder to resolve than work issues. From a t'ai chi perspective, you need to work with your current circumstances to find balance: it is an evolution that is needed, and not a revolution.

In order to deal with difficult situations involving those close to you, you can apply the t'ai chi principles of yielding and appropriateness. This means relaxing the ego-driven need always to be right, and giving way on issues where conflict would not be helpful. Just doing this will start to defuse the tension between yourself and others, and make it much more likely that both sides can find common ground. This does not mean being weak or a pushover, any more than yielding in push hands implies weakness, but it is all about appropriateness of response. When it is appropriate to stand your ground and "fight", then from an energetic standpoint you are working with the flow of the Tao and are much more likely to succeed. And because you have not overreacted to every challenge, your "opponent" knows that you are now serious about achieving your aim. This naturally engenders respect. This principle can be applied in all your dealings with other people, whenever there is the potential for some form of conflict.

DIET

An individual's diet is a major factor in achieving balanced health. Western medicine fully acknowledges this, but the Chinese medical view of diet is incredibly sophisticated, as it takes into account both the physical and the energetic properties of all foods, as well as the timing of meals and cooking methods. A full examination of Chinese dietary theory would require an entire book, but by applying some of the key principles you can help yourself regain and maintain good health.

Foods are categorized according to whether they are predominantly yin (cooling) or yang (heating); nourishing of blood or chi; causing "damp" and "phlegm" to form or disperse within the body; and which internal organs they most affect. An optimum diet is one that contains a balance of yin and yang foods, does not promote dampness or phlegm, and nourishes blood and chi. Steaming is a yin method of cooking. Boiling is more yang, grilling or baking more so, and frying is extremely yang, so you can affect the yin/yang balance of a specific food by the method of cooking.

While it is best to consult a Chinese medical practitioner to find out exactly what foods would most benefit you individually, there are a few general rules about what to avoid. Foods that promote phlegm, such as dairy foods, are best avoided, as well as foods that encourage dampness to form in the body, such as yeast (and therefore beer), heavily fried food of any sort, and wheat. This is especially relevant if you live in a damp climate. Fried food is also very "hot", however, and this can cause problems of internal heat if you live in a warm climate. In general, very spicy food should be avoided for the same reason. Heavily processed food should not be eaten as, apart from the chemical additives, the living chi energy of the food is diminished by the processing. Microwave cooking of food also disrupts chi.

Overall, a diet very much like that recommended by Western nutritionists is fine, with the exception of cold raw foods such as salads, or excessive amounts of raw fruit, which are seen as harmful to the transformative function of the spleen. Vegetables should be lightly cooked or steamed.

Below Food is truly your foundation, physically and energetically. A nutritious and balanced diet is a solid foundation for a long, healthy and happy life.

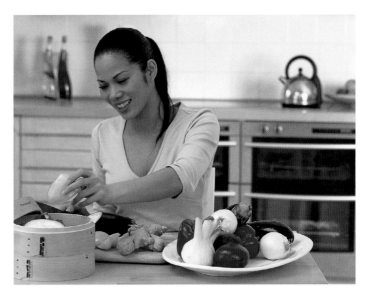

The Chinese often put ginger with steamed vegetables, as its gently warming yang nature balances the cooling, yin nature of the vegetables. Chicken is considered a well-balanced foodstuff, nourishing chi and being fairly neutral in terms of yin/yang. Chicken also nourishes the spleen, which is key to absorbing the energy of food. Beef is considered yang, and can generate internal heat in the body. This may be appropriate for a person who is internally "cold", but not for a person who is "hot". It is a good blood tonic, and this may be useful for many women who tend towards "blood deficiency" due to their menstrual cycle. If you are a vegetarian, blood-nourishing vegetables such as beetroot and spinach should be included in your diet.

The timing and regularity of meals is also seen as important. The ideal is a main meal some time between 7am and 11am, the period when the stomach and spleen are most energetically active. Following that, smaller meals can be eaten during the day, but only light snacks in the evening. This is because stomach and spleen energy is at its lowest ebb at night, and a large meal will not be properly transformed; the spleen can become "bogged down" and unhealthy weight gain may follow. A large meal late at night can also result in disturbed sleep. This accords with the principle that you should eat "breakfast like a king, lunch like a rich man, and dinner like a pauper". Achieving a balanced diet can help you resolve even deep-seated health issues, especially when combined with Chinese medical treatment and personal chi practice.

Below The early part of the night is particularly important for replenishing your yin energy.

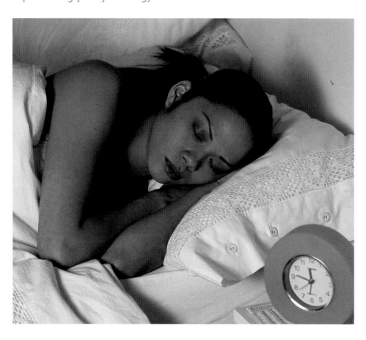

SLEEP

Proper amounts of restful sleep are essential to your well-being; what constitutes restful sleep and how to achieve it is not always so obvious.

Just as eating meals late at night can disturb your sleep, drinking alcohol at night can have the same effect – in Chinese medical terms, it can disturb the shen, or spirit. Mental tension is an obvious factor in insomnia: from a Taoist perspective it is the result of (and causes) energy becoming stuck in the brain, over-energizing it and causing repetitive and excessive thinking, with the mind "whirling around". This is a condition that is particularly prevalent in those who spend the day involved in mental work. The brain becomes so energized that mental activity refuses to subside when it is time to sleep. In chi gung terms, this is the result of energy not dropping from the brain to the lower tantien and feet. A simple but highly effective remedy is to roll your ankles at least 50 times in each direction – this brings your chi down to your feet and allows your brain to de-energize and calm down. Standing practice and gentle t'ai chi practice before bedtime also help enormously.

It is important to allow a winding-down period before going to bed. Try to avoid any mental work late at night, including the taking in of new information such as reading and watching the television immediately before bedtime. Listening to music, massage (especially of the feet), a warm bath – all these can allow your mind to settle prior to sleep, helping to counter insomnia. It is also very important, in terms of the natural energetic cycle of day and night, that you go to sleep before midnight if possible.

TAOIST SEXUAL PRACTICE

The Taoists have a matter-of fact attitude to sex: they see it simply as one of life's natural activities and do not impose any moral judgements upon it. Some people are more interested in sexual activity, some less – this is a personal preference. Where the Taoists do distinguish sex from other activities is in relation to energy: it is probably the most energetically "alive" experience that most people have. As a result of this it is seen as a very powerful practice, where those taking part can work with the strong energies involved to heal, release blockages and tensions in any of their energetic bodies, develop and strengthen their energy and, of course, enhance sexual pleasure. A range of techniques can help to achieve this; some are concerned more with the physical and chi levels, and some with meditation.

All the Taoist nei gung practices that underlie t'ai chi are applicable during sex. Sexual chi gung is very powerful and best approached gently. As with anything else, excessive

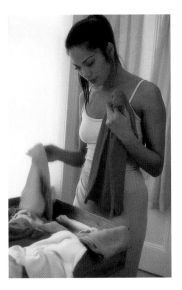

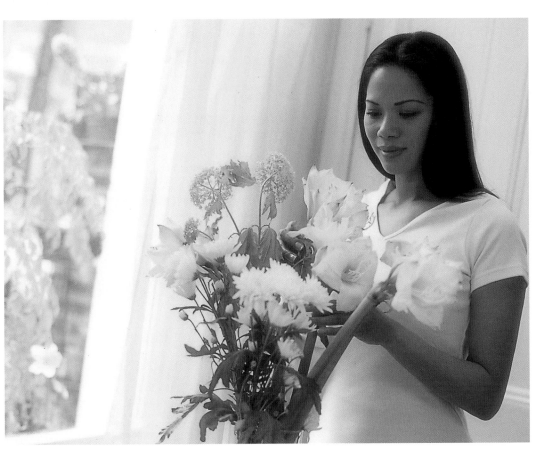

Above Every object has its own energetic quality and can influence your energy. Colours can strongly influence your mental and emotional state.

Right Making your living space full of light and life will have a corresponding effect on you.

activity leads to imbalance. What constitutes excess depends on the individual; as a general rule if you feel energetically "drained" rather than just relaxed after sex, it may mean activity has been excessive, or your approach to it has not been sufficiently relaxed.

EXERCISE

The best exercise you can engage in is t'ai chi or another Taoist internal art, but in fact, any gentle exercise is beneficial, helping to eliminate stagnation of chi and blood, and keeping your body flexible. Over-strenuous exercise can be energetically draining, and damaging to your body. If you do other exercise, especially weights, do it with relaxation. T'ai chi is ideal because it is not only a gentle physical exercise, but also works directly with your energy and mind. The body abhors inactivity – energy and blood stagnate, and the joints and tissues stiffen and contract. Constant gentle movement is ideal, and is one of the keys to longevity.

DRUGS

Just as the Taoists do not form moral judgements about sex, they also do not ascribe any moral attributes to drugs, but consider them to be substances that have a strong effect on your energy and mind. So-called recreational drugs are not considered "evil", they just do not bring the user any benefits, and cause greater or lesser degrees of harm to the body, energy and mind. Because drugs do not promote balance, they are not considered useful, and are best avoided. Caffeine and alcohol are seen to be less harmful, and acceptable as part of a balanced lifestyle. Nicotine is not considered a useful substance.

OTHER FACTORS

Many aspects of your life, such as whether you maintain clean and tidy living spaces, what sort of clothes you wear, and your general mental attitudes towards yourself and others, can have a profound effect on your health and well-being. A home full of clutter and mess invokes scattered and disordered energy, and this will have a corresponding effect on you, in terms of both your internal world and the things that happen to you. Similarly, a dirty and neglected home will attract negative energies that will promote illness, both physical and emotional. Conversely, a clean, ordered home, full of life, will encourage a positive energy response, as well as simply making you feel more cheerful.

Wearing drab, worn or dirty clothes can also have a negative effect in terms of the energies you attract. This does not mean dressing like a harlequin – simply introducing some life and colour into your wardrobe. It can also be beneficial to consider which colours have a positive effect on your energy and mind, and dress accordingly. Experiment to find out for yourself how different colours can affect you.

How you behave towards other people determines not only how other people treat you but invokes a subtle energetic response from the universe as a whole. The phrase "Do unto others as you would have done to yourself" sums this up.

You should try to make every aspect of your life reflect the way you would like to live – bringing a sense of balance, liveliness and joy into all aspects of your day-to-day life. This means nurturing and respecting yourself, being aware of your inherent self-worth and celebrating it every day.

The Short Form

The short form is shown here from start to finish, it is best used as a quick reference once you have become familar with the positions.

Commencement

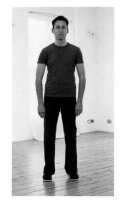 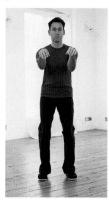 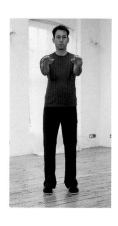 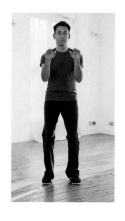 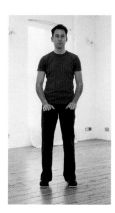 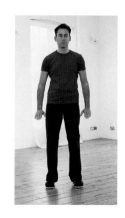

Raise Hands

Play the Lute

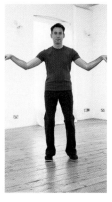 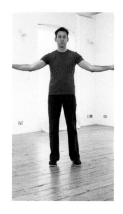 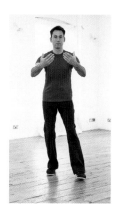 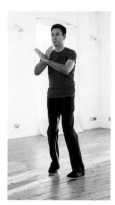 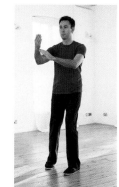

Grasp Sparrow's Tail

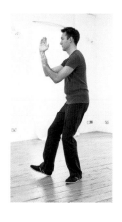 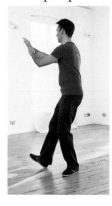 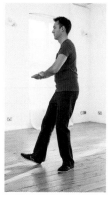 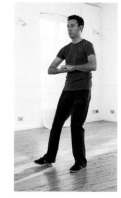 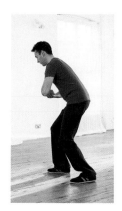 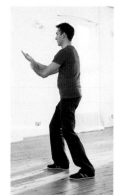

Single Whip

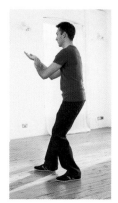 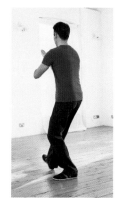 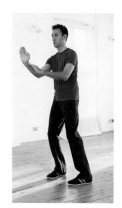 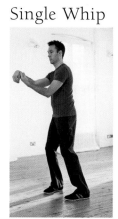 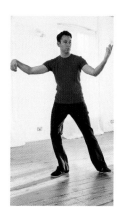 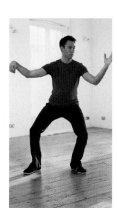

Diagonal Flying / Hold Ball

Yin Release / Shoulder Stroke

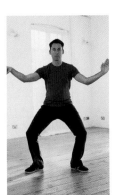 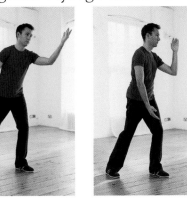 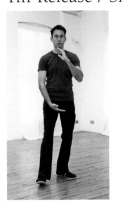 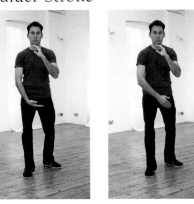 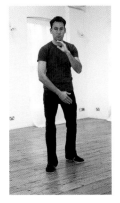

Elbow Strike / Wrist Strike

White Crane Spreads its Wings

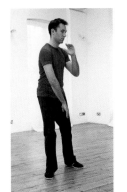 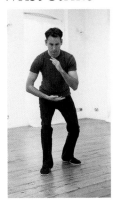 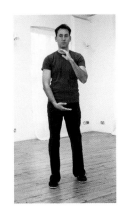 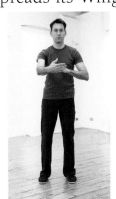 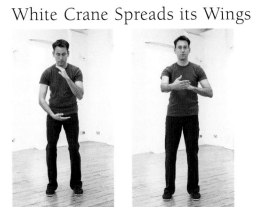

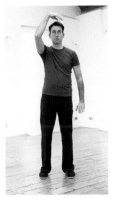 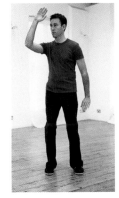 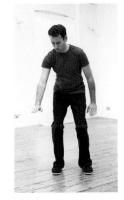 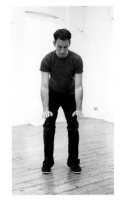 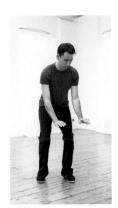 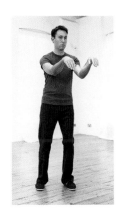

Brush Knee and Twist Step

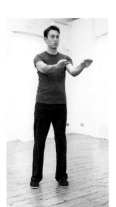 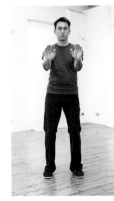 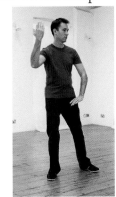 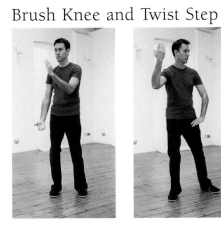 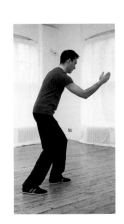 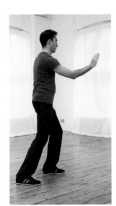

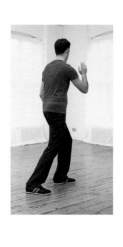 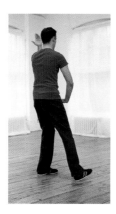 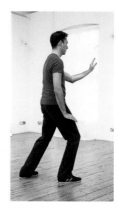 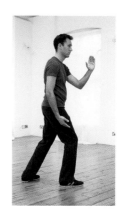 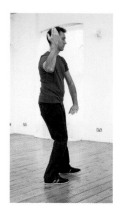 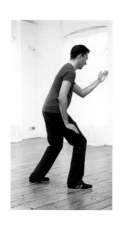

Needle at Sea Bottom

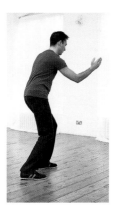 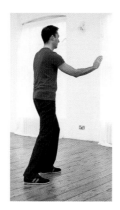 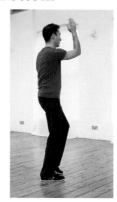 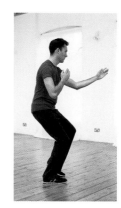 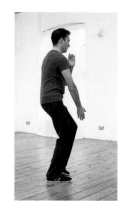 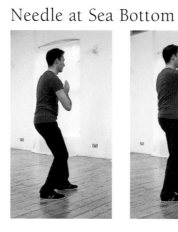

Fan Through the Back   Turn and Chop with Back of F

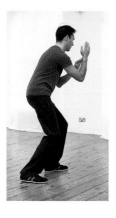 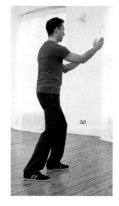 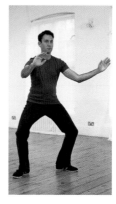 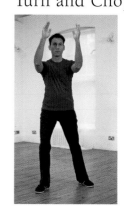 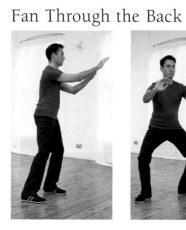 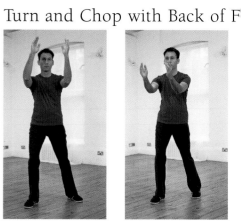

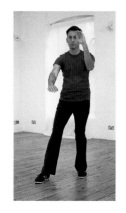 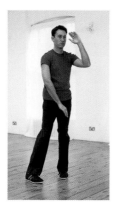 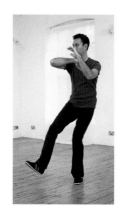 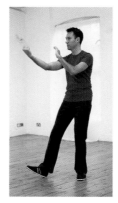 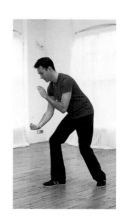 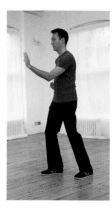

Parry and Punch

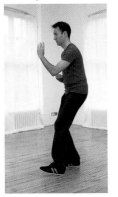 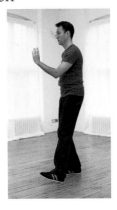 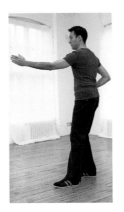 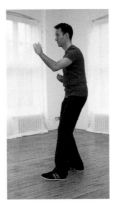 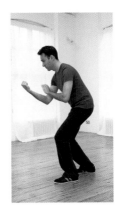 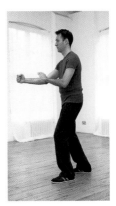

Close up and Step Forward

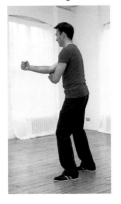 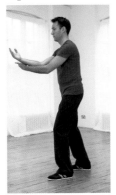 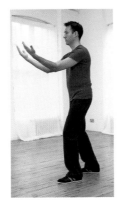 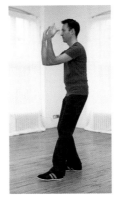 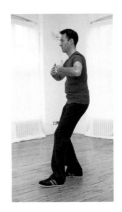 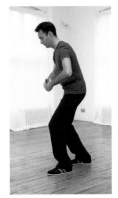

Tiger and Leopard Spring to Mountain

Closing

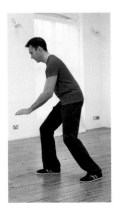 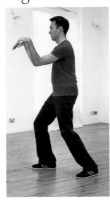 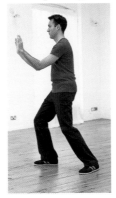 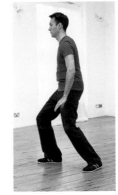 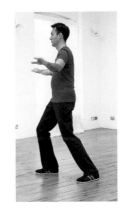 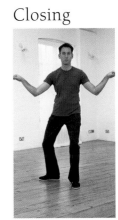

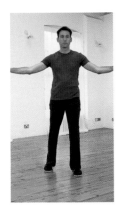 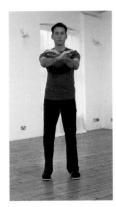 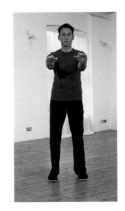 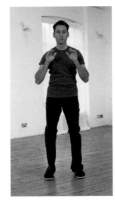 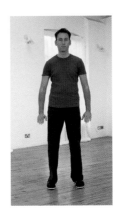 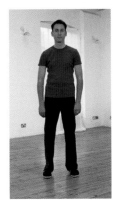

Choosing a Teacher, School and Style

This book is designed to kindle your interest in t'ai chi and the Taoist internal arts, and kick-start your practice. It provides you with usable methods to start learning t'ai chi principles and form, as well as serving as a reference for your continued development as you progress. However, the importance of finding a good teacher cannot be exaggerated. T'ai chi is a complex movement art, and it is possible to take wrong turns in your t'ai chi path without even realizing it. A competent teacher can show you the way and correct any mistakes, to help you make the most of the time and effort that you put into learning and practising t'ai chi. In addition, working with a teacher who has developed their own chi will have a direct effect on your energy, greatly accelerating your progress.

FINDING A TEACHER

Finding a good teacher is not particularly difficult if you know what to look for and where to look for it. The most obvious consideration is who is teaching t'ai chi in your area, within easy travel distance. Gather all the information you can on t'ai chi schools and teachers in your region. The internet is increasingly the best source of contacts for this, but you may also find flyers, brochures or posters

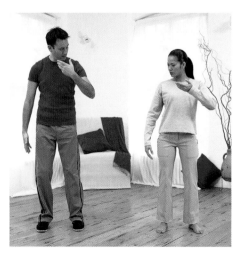

locally, and there may be tuition in your local health or sports centre. Separate out the schools and teachers that claim to teach one of the acknowledged major styles of t'ai chi. Good t'ai chi teachers generally emphasize their links with the major lineages, rather than creating their own "brand-name" of t'ai chi. Look for direct links with the major lineages of t'ai chi and well-known lineage masters of past and present. This makes it much more likely that your teacher will be in possession of genuine knowledge and skill, which they can then pass on to you.

CHOOSING A SCHOOL

Having found some likely candidates, take your time before committing to any school. Call ahead and visit several schools and watch both beginner's and intermediate classes. If a teacher refuses to let you watch a class before joining, this is not a good sign. Observe the atmosphere in the classes. Are the students enjoying themselves? Are they friendly and cooperative with one another, rather than competitive and overly serious? Is the teacher relaxed and easy-going yet also confident and commanding in their teaching style? What sort of feeling do you get from the teacher's energy? Is their energy relaxed yet full?

Talk to both the main teacher and some of the students. Do not be afraid to ask about the teaching style and methods. Ask about some of the principles and nei gung aspects of t'ai chi that are in this book. These concepts should be familiar to any good t'ai chi teacher. Ask the teacher who their main teacher is or was. Ask the students how long they have trained with that school and whether they have benefited and progressed.

Some schools are more martial in emphasis, some are more health and

meditation oriented. The best are both, with everything being done in a relaxed and non-aggressive way.

Most good schools expect their students to show appropriate respect towards the teacher and the material being taught. However, a guru worship atmosphere is not appropriate.

The cost of classes should not be your major consideration – if you find a good school, you will certainly get value for money. Very cheap or free classes, or those in subsidized health clubs rarely yield the inner benefits of t'ai chi. Good teachers simply do not have to teach for free – they attract and retain paying students.

CHOOSING A STYLE

Which style of t'ai chi you choose will most likely depend on which teacher or school you choose. If you are lucky enough to have a choice of good schools of different styles, then try a short course in each style and make your decision based on which style instinctively feels right for you. Good t'ai chi is good t'ai chi in whatever style, so quality of teaching should come first; style is a relative second.

PROGRESSING

Once you have chosen a t'ai chi school, stick with it for at least six months. Learning t'ai chi can take a little perseverance, and initial frustrations may not be the fault of the school or teacher but simply part of the process. If after that time you are still convinced that a different school would suit you better, you may wish to change. As you progress, the school that you started with may cater for this, or you may find that you need to seek more advanced tuition elsewhere. Studying privately in one-to-one sessions with a good teacher is also an excellent adjunct to whatever group classes you are taking.

Useful Contacts and Further Reading

CHIWORKS
Taoist Internal Arts
Chinese Medical Therapy
London, UK
Contact: Andrew Popovic
Web: www.chiworks.org
Email: info@chiworks.org
Tel: +44 (0)7939 663 082

B.K. FRANTZIS ENERGY ARTS
Fairfax, CA, USA
Web: www.energyarts.com
Email: admin@energyarts.com
Tel: +1 415 454 5243

JOHN DING INTERNATIONAL
ACADEMY OF T'AI CHI CHUAN
London, UK
Web: www.taichiwl.demon.co.uk
Email: JDIATCC@taichiwl.demon.co.uk
Tel: +44 (0)20 8502 9307

REAL TAOISM
Taoist Life Arts
Unit 9
170 Brick Lane
London E1 6RU
Tel: 020 7247 1399

T'AI CHI UNION FOR GREAT BRITAIN
Web: www.taichiunion.com
Email: secretary@taichiunion.com
Tel: +44 (0)141 810 3482

T'AI CHI FINDER
Web: www.taichifinder.co.uk

T'AI CHI MAGAZINE
International monthly publication
Wayfarer Publications
P.O. Box 39938
Los Angeles, CA 90039
USA
(800) 888-9119 toll-free
fax: 323-665-1627

WORLDWIDE T'AI CHI CHUAN
www.middx.org.uk/gordo/2tai_links.html
www.scheele.org/lee/tcclinks.html

WORLD T'AI CHI AND CHI GUNG DAY
www.worldtaichiday.com

FURTHER READING

Opening the Energy Gates of Your Body: Gain Lifelong Vitality
Bruce Kumar Frantzis

Relaxing into Your Being: The Water Method of Taoist Meditation Series, Volume I
Bruce Kumar Frantzis

The Great Stillness: The Water Method of Taoist Meditation Series, Volume II
Bruce Kumar Frantzis

The Power of Internal Martial Arts: Combat Secrets of Ba Gua, Tai Chi and Hsing-I
Bruce Kumar Frantzis

Cheng Tzu's Thirteen Treatises on T'ai Chi Ch'uan
Cheng Man-ch'ing

Tai Chi Touchstones: Yang Family Secret Transmissions
Douglas Wyle

Tai Chi Chuan for Health and Self-defense
T. T. Liang

Steal my Art: Memoirs of a 100 year-

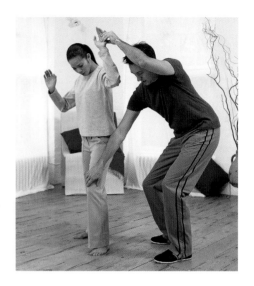

old T'ai Chi Master
T. T. Liang, Stuart Alve Olson

Tao Te Ching: Lao-zu's Tao Te Ching
Lao-zi, Red Pine

Tao Te Ching: Definitive Edition
Lao Tzu, Jonathan Star

Hua Hu Ching: Later Teachings of Lao Tzu
Hua-Ching Ni

The Taoist I Ching
Thomas Cleary

The Essential Chuang-Tzu
Sam Hamill, J. P. Seaton

The Way of Chuang Tzu
Thomas Merton

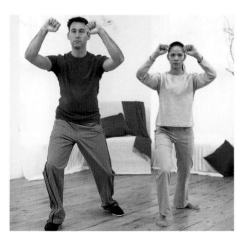

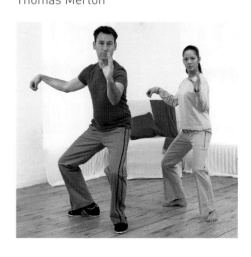

Glossary

an: push downwards
ba gua: eight trigrams
baihui: crown of head
beng chuan: crushing fist
chan ssu jin: silk-reeling energy
chi: energy
chi gung: energy work
chien: heaven
da lu: moving step push hands
fa jin: issuing power
fu: yang organs
heng chuan: crossing fist
hsin: heart-mind
hsing-i: mind-form fist
huiyin: perineum
i: intent
jan: yielding
ji: press
jiao: lower organs
jing: essence
jou: elbow stroke
kao: shoulder stroke
ko: controlling cycle

kou: tiger's mouth
kung fu: skill
kwa: inguinal area at front of pelvis
lan: merging
laogung: centre of the palm
lieh: split
lu: roll back
ming men: bright gate/gate of life
moxa: mugwort
nei gung: internal work
nei jia: internal arts
nien: merging
pao chuan: pounding fist
pao twi: cannon fist
peng: ward off
pi chuan: splitting fist
san ti: hsing-i standing posture
shen: spirit
sheng: generating cycle
soong: unbound
suei: magnetizing
tantien: body's energy centre
ting jin: listening energy

tsai: pull down
tsuan chuan: drilling fist
tsuan jin: drilling energy
tui na: Chinese massage
tui shou: push hands
wei chi: protective energy
wei: external
wu chi: ultimate emptiness
wushu: fighting method
yongquan: Bubbling Well point, hollow in ball of foot
zang: yin organs
zhan zhuang: standing like a tree

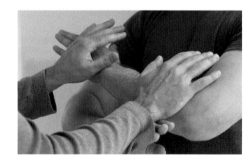

Acknowledgements

Above all, a debt of gratitude is owed to the generation of masters who have now passed, for opening the great secrets of their culture to benefit the rest of the world.

First I would like to thank my Taoist masters, especially my main teacher Lineage Master Bruce Kumar Frantzis, for his many teachings and powerful transmissions of the Taoist internal arts, including his transmission of the Wu style of t'ai chi. I would also like to thank Lineage Master John Ding for his training in the Yang style of t'ai chi and his invaluable input. Thanks also to Chris Chappell for his insightful instruction and advice over the years.

To my Tibetan Dzogchen masters, especially Namkhai Norbu Rinpoche; words are truly insufficient to express my gratitude for your teachings.

A special thanks goes to my family, friends and students for their enthusiasm, encouragement and support for this book. I hope it serves to inspire many people to take up and enjoy this wonderful art.

Finally, many thanks to Joanne Rippin of Anness Publishing, for her patience and skill in managing the book, to Clare Park for her excellent photography, and to Adrian Hope-Lewis for standing in as a cheerful and willing training partner.

Anness Publishing would like to thank the following agencies for the use of their images:
Bridgeman Art Library: pp12, 14, Corbis: pp7, 8, 13, 16, 18, 19 top, 20, 22, 23, 44 (both), 112, 113.

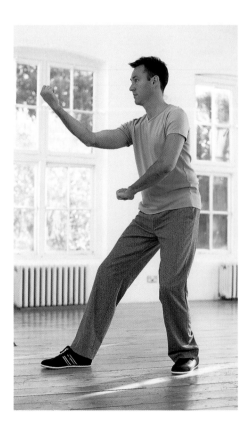

Index

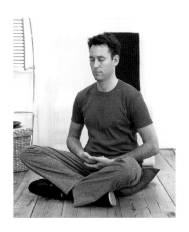

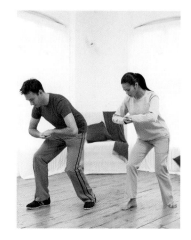

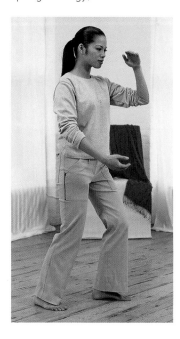